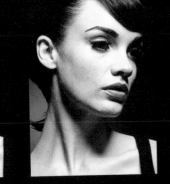
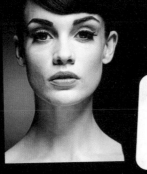

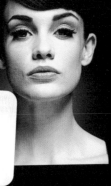
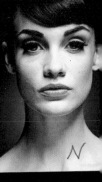
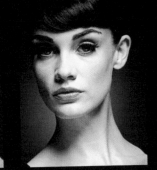
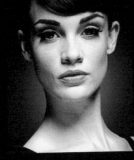
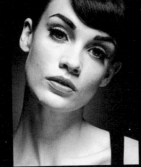
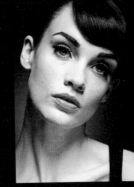
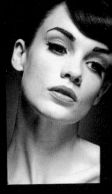
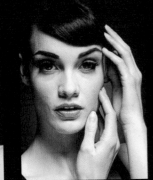
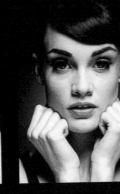
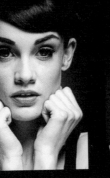
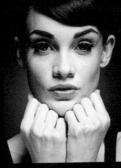
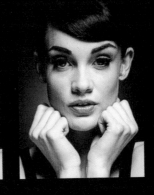
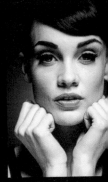
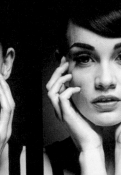
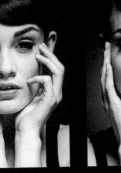
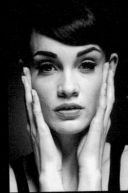
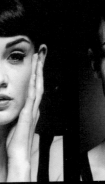
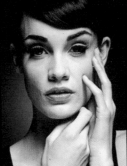
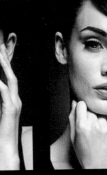
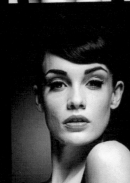
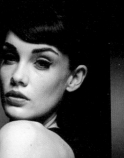
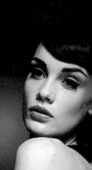

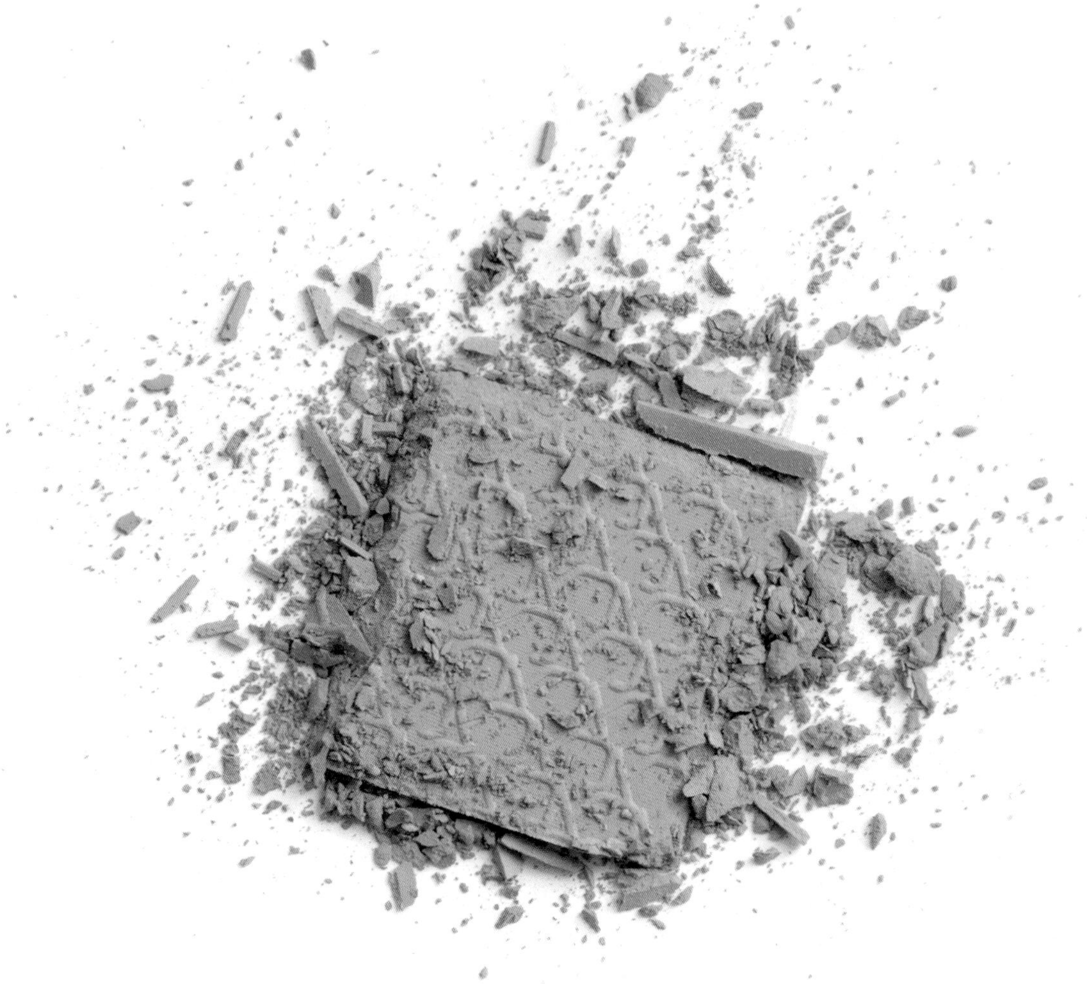

JEMMA KIDD MAKE-UP SECRETS

Photographer **Vikki Grant**   Text **Zia Mattocks**

St. Martin's Press
New York

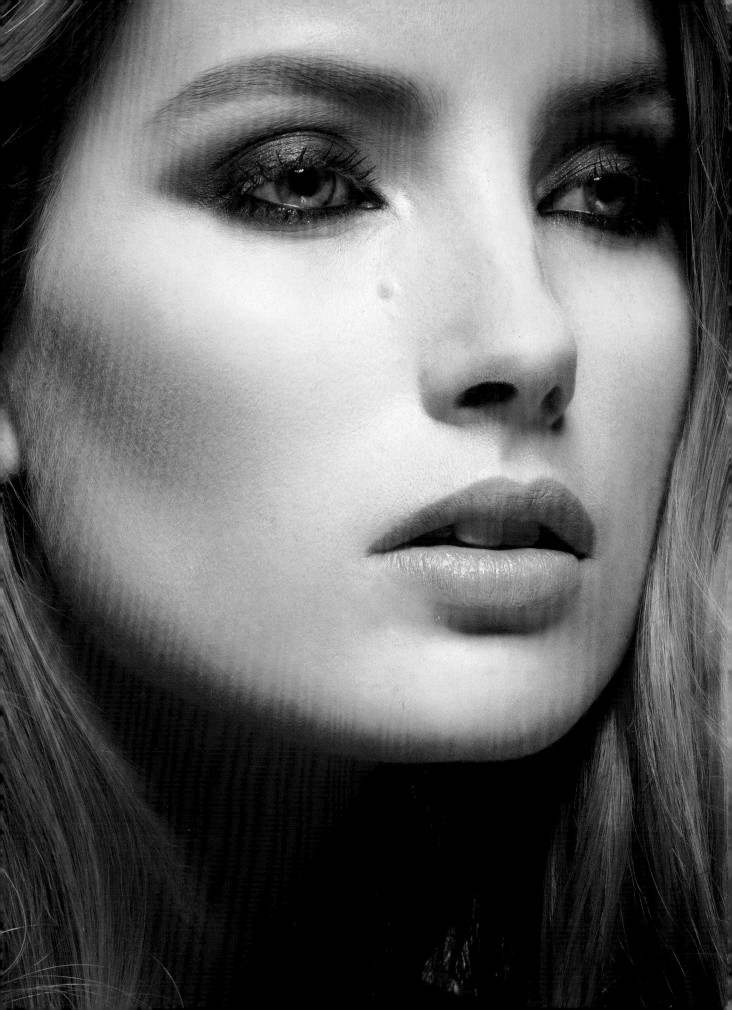

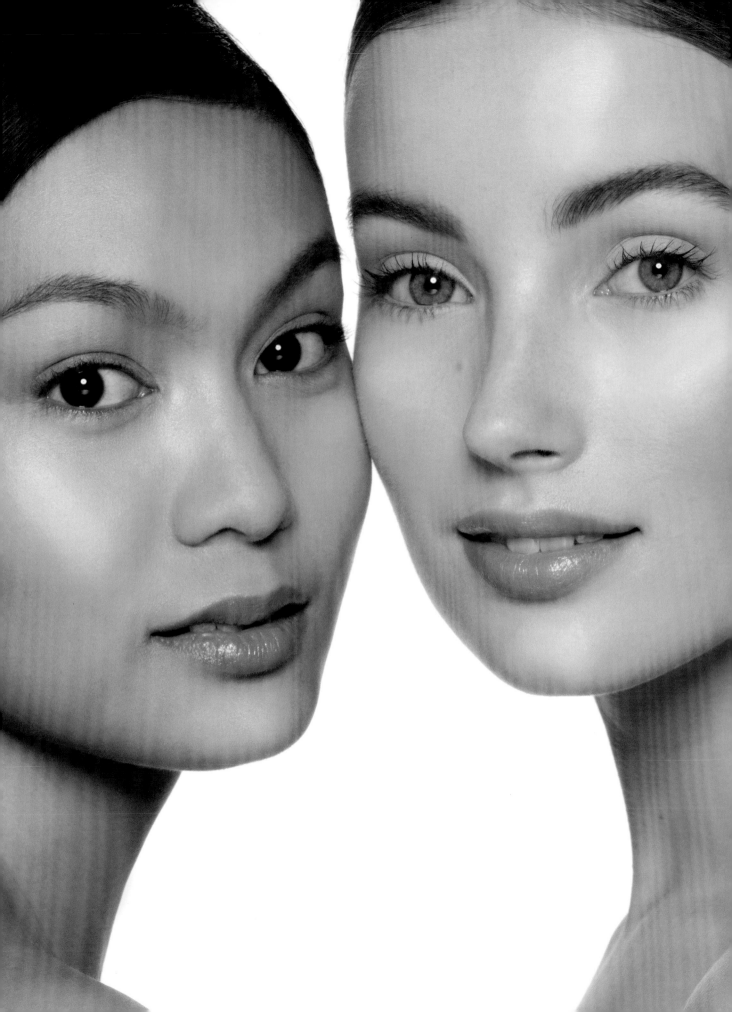

CONTENTS

Introduction 6 ✳ The power of make-up 8

PART 1 MAKING MAKE-UP WORK FOR YOU

PART 2 PROBLEM SOLVER

JEMMA KIDD MAKE-UP SECRETS.
Text copyright © 2012 by Jemma Kidd.
Photography, design, and layout copyright
© 2012 by Jacqui Small. All rights reserved.
Printed in China. For information, address
St. Martin's Press, 175 Fifth Avenue,
New York, N.Y. 10010.

www.stmartins.com

The written instructions, photographs,
designs, patterns, and projects in this
volume are intended for personal use
of the reader and may be reproduced
for that purpose only.

Library of Congress Cataloging-in-
Publication Data Available Upon Request

ISBN 978-1-250-01086-5

First U.S. Edition: November 2012

10 9 8 7 6 5 4 3 2 1

INTRODUCTION

When I was asked to write a new book, I nearly jumped for joy. I had the most wonderful time creating my first book, Jemma Kidd Make-Up Masterclass. It was the product of all my industry knowledge and what I had been teaching in the make-up school for years. In this book I wanted to go in-depth into all the problem-solving tricks and techniques that I have learned over the years. I looked at everything from skin tones to eye shapes, and thought hard about what women find challenging about make-up and the beauty problems they come up against every day. No two women's faces, eyes, and lips are the same. Eye shape, in particular, is something to consider and I wanted to demonstrate the different ways of applying make-up to achieve the most flattering effects. I also wanted to address many other beauty issues that I know concern the majority of women—from acne to aging—so I have brought in two friends to share their specialist knowledge, skincare guru Sarah Chapman and nutritionist Petronella Ravenshear. I have consulted both of them for years for their invaluable advice, and both are experts in their fields. Through years of trying to find the answer to perfect skin, I have realized that it's not all about what you put on the skin. There is no magic cream that diminishes wrinkles—trust me, if there was, I would have mortgaged my house to buy it. But what you put inside your body, together with how you care for your skin, can make a big difference.

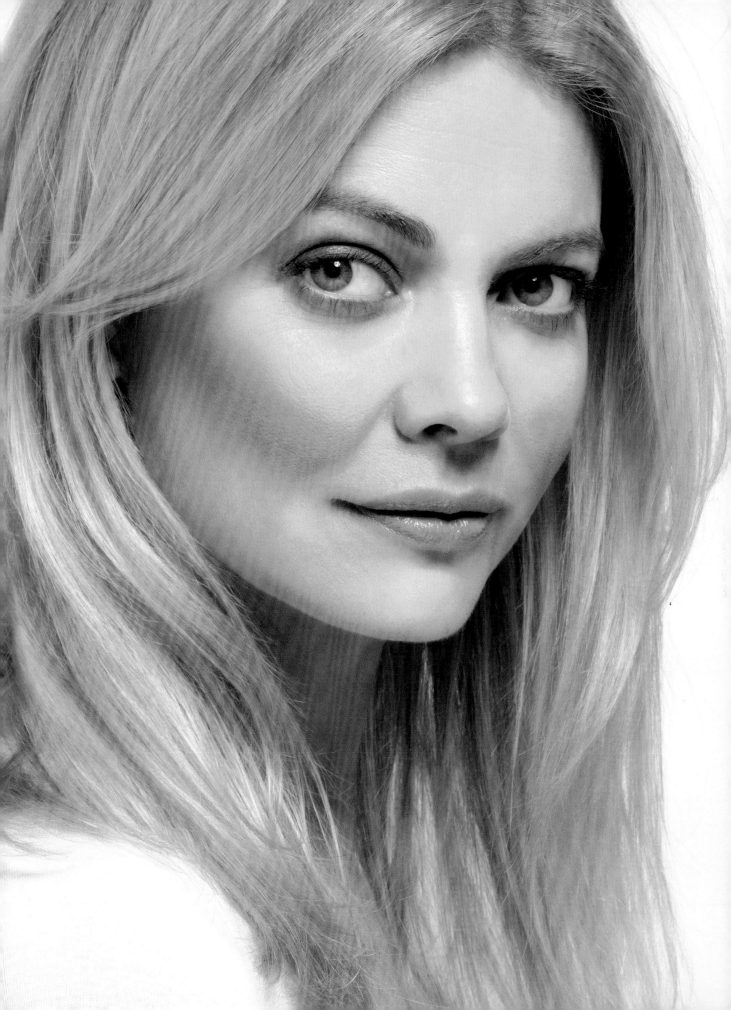

THE POWER OF MAKE-UP

Make-up is so much more than a bit of color on the face. Used in the right way, it gives women the ability to enhance and emphasize their best features and play down their least favorite aspects of their appearance.

Make-up can perfect skin, restore a youthful glow, disguise blemishes and undereye shadows, give the illusion of sharply defined cheekbones, make eyes look bigger, noses look smaller, and lips look fuller. On an emotional level, wearing make-up lifts the mood and gives confidence—if you look good, you feel good, and vice versa.

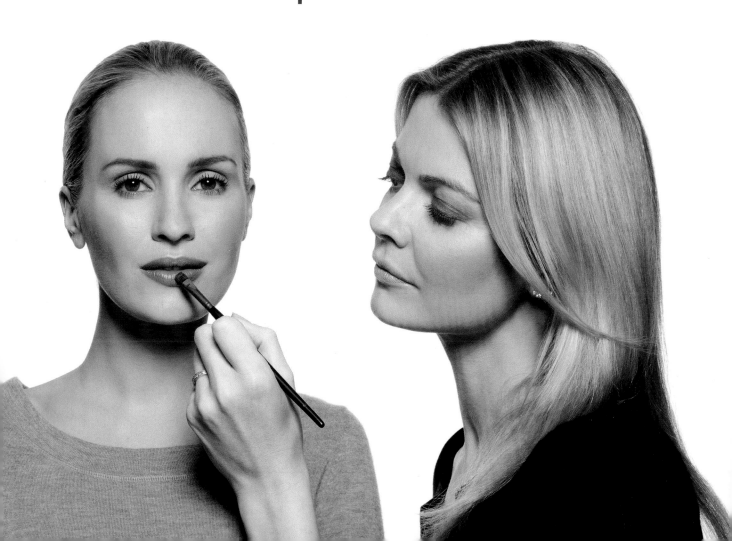

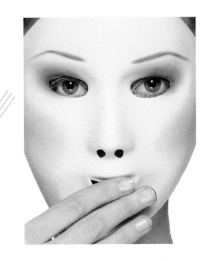

> *Make-up may not be life-changing, but it can certainly be face-changing.*

Running the make-up school is a massive source of inspiration for me, as I discover the beauty concerns and product wish-lists of my clients. So many women tell me they are stuck in a make-up rut and comfortable with a certain way of doing things. As a make-up artist, I'm not intimidated by make-up and am willing to experiment with it, so it is interesting for me to have a constant reminder that techniques I think are easy, are actually things that a lot of women consider difficult.

I wanted to demonstrate problem-solving techniques for some of the most frequently encountered issues, as well as illustrate how different applications of the same product— eyeliner, for instance—can change the face, producing effects ranging from subtle and natural to extreme and dramatic. This is one aspect of make-up that really excites me. I also wanted to show how to create modern timeless looks and wearable fashion looks, which are both things I am asked about all the time.

The cosmetics industry is continually evolving and the best modern formulations are not just about color or even staying power, but have the combined benefits of anti-aging and skin-conditioning ingredients, too. Natural skincare and mineral make-up are becoming increasingly mainstream, as there is more awareness about the potential effects of what we absorb into our bodies through the skin. As a response to these advances, both hybrid and mineral make-up have become important features of my brand.

It's never too late to discover new products, learn new make-up tricks, or find different ways to enhance your features or care for your skin. The main thing is to have fun experimenting—try a different color, texture, or technique, or take a whole new approach—and keep in mind that make-up shouldn't be a mask to hide behind, but a tool to let you reveal the best version of you.

MAKE-UP IN CONTEXT

\# Always consider the overall finished look.

\# If you're wearing a sexy outfit, you might want to match that with vampy make-up.

\# If you're dressing low-key, keep your make-up natural and fresh with a soft lipstick or gloss, a simple wash of nude eyeshadow, and mascara.

\# Balance your look: wear a punchy lip color with just mascara on your eyes, or pair rock-chick smoky eyes with tinted balm on your lips.

\# If you want to wear a full face of make-up, choose tones that work together so they don't clash—likewise with your clothes.

MAKE-UP MUST-HAVES

I can't live without …

foundation and concealer ✳ skin illuminator
peachy/apricot blush ✳ tweezers
eyelash curlers ✳ mascara ✳ tinted lip balm

I asked all my lovely followers on Twitter what make-up they take out with them on a night out. Lipstick/gloss, mascara, eyeliner, concealer, and powder all came above foundation, blotting paper, bronzer, blush, and eyeshadow.

1

MAKING MAKE-UP WORK FOR YOU

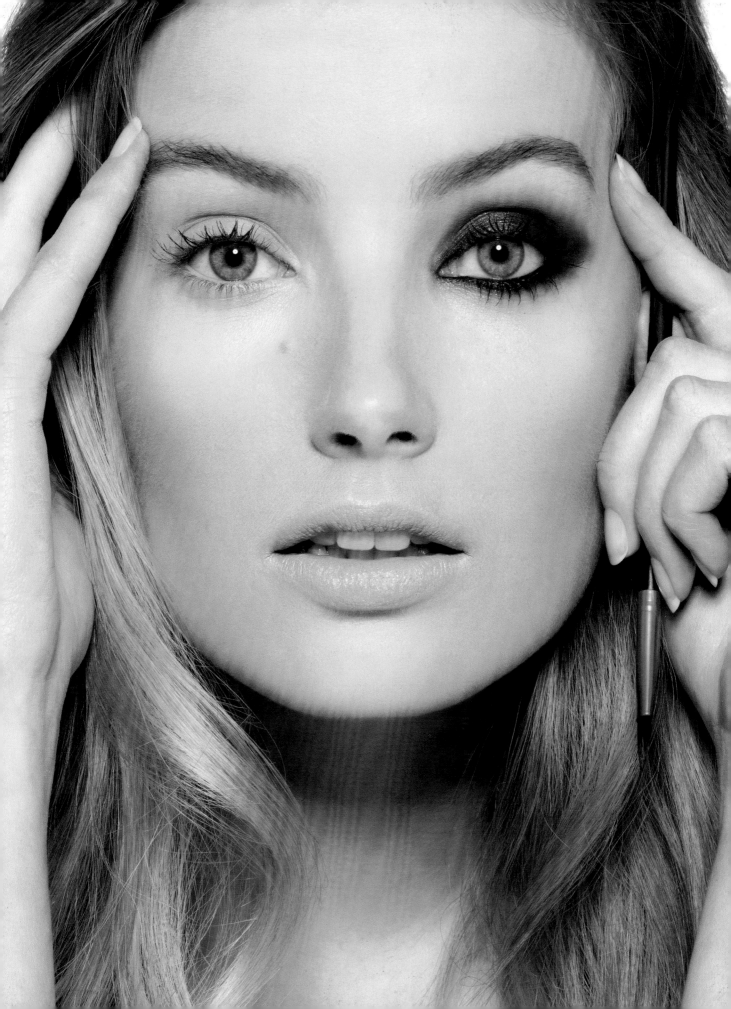

My philosophy is that make-up
is there to enhance, not hide
behind—it should make you
look like you, but better.

naturally
beautiful

We are lucky enough, these days, to have
incredible products at our disposal that make
us look good all year round, whatever age we
are and whatever our skin is like. There are
formulations to boost radiance, smooth fine
lines, minimize pores, and even out skin tone—
and the results are subtle and very natural.
Make-up is a powerful tool that can create
definition, symmetry, depth, and shadow; it can
sculpt and contour your face or take 10 years
off you. Using just one or two products can alter
how you feel about yourself within moments,
and if you have confidence in your looks, you
automatically look even better.

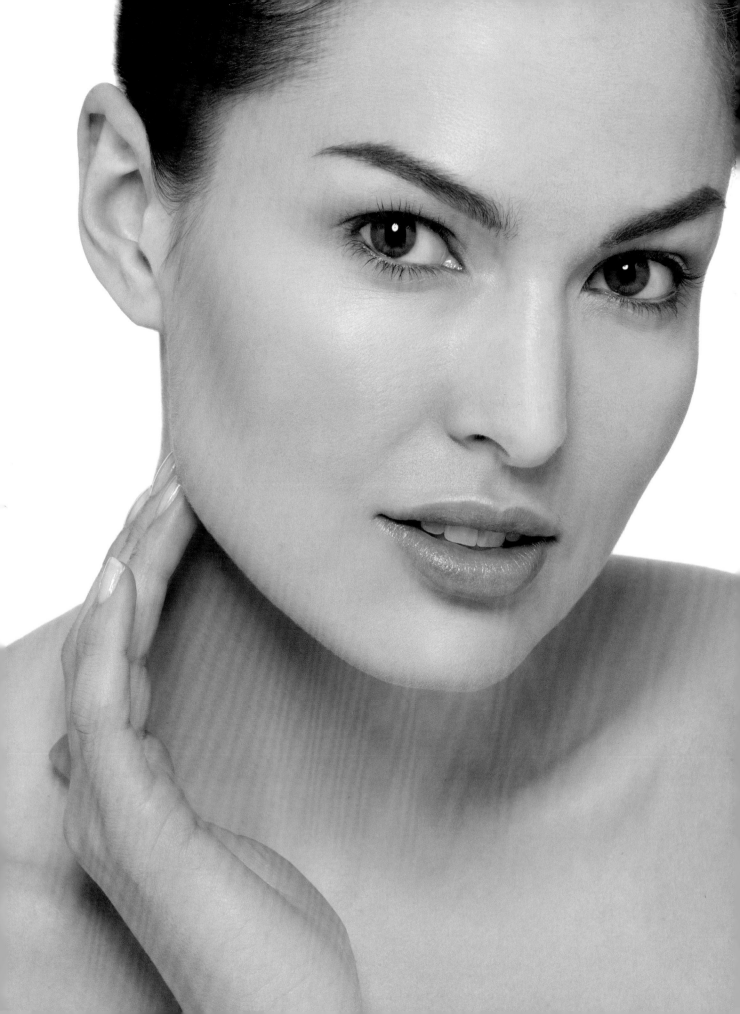

BRING OUT THE BEST "YOU"

The first step to good make-up is to identify your best features. It is then easy to learn ways to make the most of them—as well as to disguise any perceived flaws.

Women often find it hard to acknowledge the good things about the way they look. We can be far too critical, dwelling on the negatives, when we should be focusing on our good points. Learn to look at yourself objectively, so that you can understand your face and accept what's good about your appearance. There are always going to be things you don't like. I've always hated my nose, but I like my smile. You might dislike your square jaw, but love your eyes. Once you've learned to see your attractive qualities, you can learn to enhance them and make them the focal points.

Beauty comes from within: if you feel beautiful, you look beautiful.

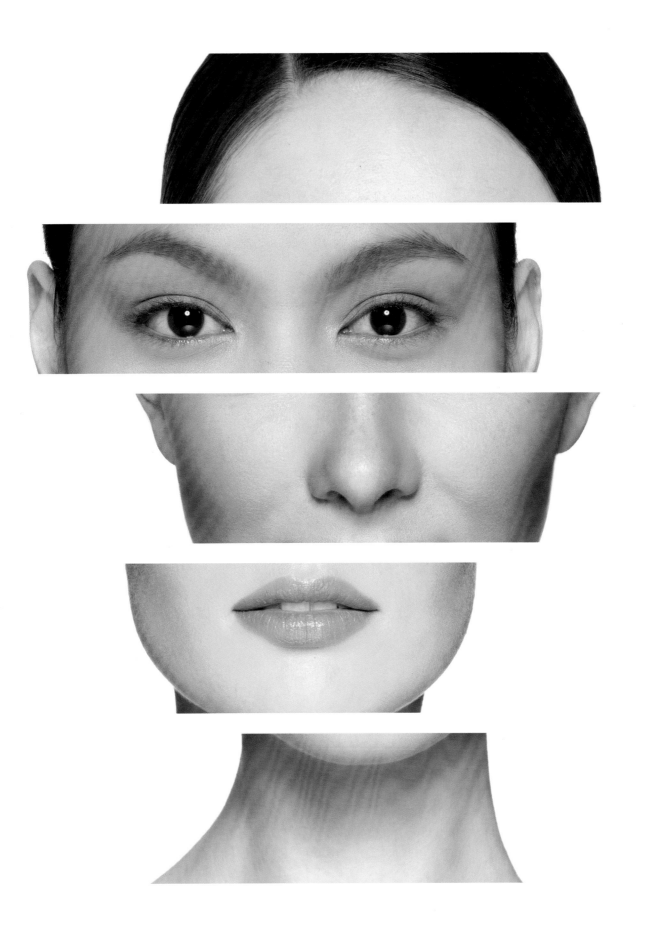

skin secrets

It all starts with the skin. The largest organ in the body, our skin is the true indicator of how we are feeling inside. It shows the first signs of aging, puffiness, dehydration, sun spots, flakiness, broken capillaries, open pores, blemishes—the list is endless. The skin on the face can be very cruel and women spend their life focusing on that area of their body, so getting this right is key.

The good news is that there are small things you can do to help—hydration, cleanliness, sleep, better nutrition, relaxation, and good grooming.

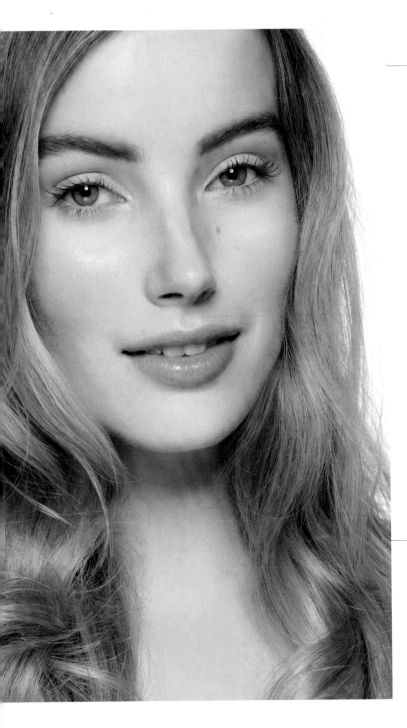

THE BOTTOM LINE

You can't expect to look great if you don't take care of yourself—it's a commitment and a dedication you need to make to yourself. If you fill your body with processed foods, alcohol, caffeine, and other toxins, then unfortunately your face will be the first place to mirror that. This isn't brain surgery, it's a simple equation.

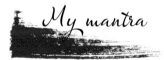

My mantra

Everything in moderation. You don't have to be an angel and it's important to enjoy yourself, but if you know you haven't been doing yourself any favors, take steps to redress the balance.

HELPFUL HINT

If you have any persistent skincare concerns, go to see a specialist and let them diagnose your skin. A dermatologist can give you a tailor-made "prescription" that could just change your life.

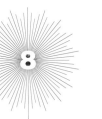

1

Eat a good diet full of fresh organic food and plenty of fiber to maintain a healthy digestive system; avoid processed or packaged food (see pages 162–7).

2

Drink at least 5 glasses (1.5 liters) of still water throughout the day (see page 160).

Top 10 ways to healthy skin

3

Get enough sleep—a good night's rest can take years off you. Magnesium oil is a great relaxant, and a warm bath with Epsom salts before bed will help you sleep.

4

Cleanse and moisturize every day. A good skincare regime, using products appropriate for your skin, will help keep it in optimum condition (see pages 154–9 and 172–3).

5

Exfoliate regularly to slough off the dead cells on the surface and encourage the rejuvenation of the skin underneath. Some very gentle exfoliators can be used daily, whereas others should only be used once or twice a week (see page 171).

6

Stress has a negative impact on the skin, so make sure you find balance in your life by having time out for yourself, in whatever way works for you. Meditation, soaking in the tub, and no phone calls or emailing after 6pm are all things that help me to unwind.

7

Exercise is good for the skin, as it aids circulation, increasing oxygen levels in the blood and speeding up the elimination of toxins. Exercising in the fresh air is even better, giving you that unmistakable healthy glow.

8

Maintenance—if you can, see a facialist once every couple of months, or whenever you feel you need it, for a really good cleanse. This is especially beneficial if you have oily skin.

9

Colonics and liver detoxes are really good for the skin, as they accelerate the elimination of toxins from your system.

10

Wear SPF on your face all year round—ideally Factor 30 in the winter and Factor 50 in the summer. This will help to prevent signs of aging.

PERFECT COMPLEXION

If you take the time to make your skin look good, you will find that often you don't need to wear much make-up at all.

Achieving perfect-looking skin is more straightforward than it sounds. Nowadays, with all the hybrid make-up that combines skincare and color, you don't have to layer your skin with numerous products.

It is important to prepare the skin properly before you start applying make-up. Spending time creating a good canvas will reap long-term benefits, as it will help keep your skin in peak condition. It will also give your make-up greater staying power.

The biggest problem I see on women—one that can be put right so easily—is redness and unevenness in skin tone. If you make addressing this your main aim, you can't go far wrong.

HOW I MAKE UP MY FACE

Everyone is different and you can adapt your regime depending on your skin, but here's what I do:

After using a gentle cleanser—anything from Dove soap to a mild cream—I apply an antioxidant serum with a high Vitamin C content and a moisturizer with SPF (Factor 30 in winter and 50 in summer). Then I neutralize any redness using my Citrus Color Corrector (see page 25). I don't like the look of too much foundation on the skin, so sometimes I just use a tinted moisturizer to balance out my skin tone. If I need more coverage, I use a light-reflecting liquid foundation.

Only wear make-up where you need it. Don't cover up good skin—if you've got it, flaunt it.

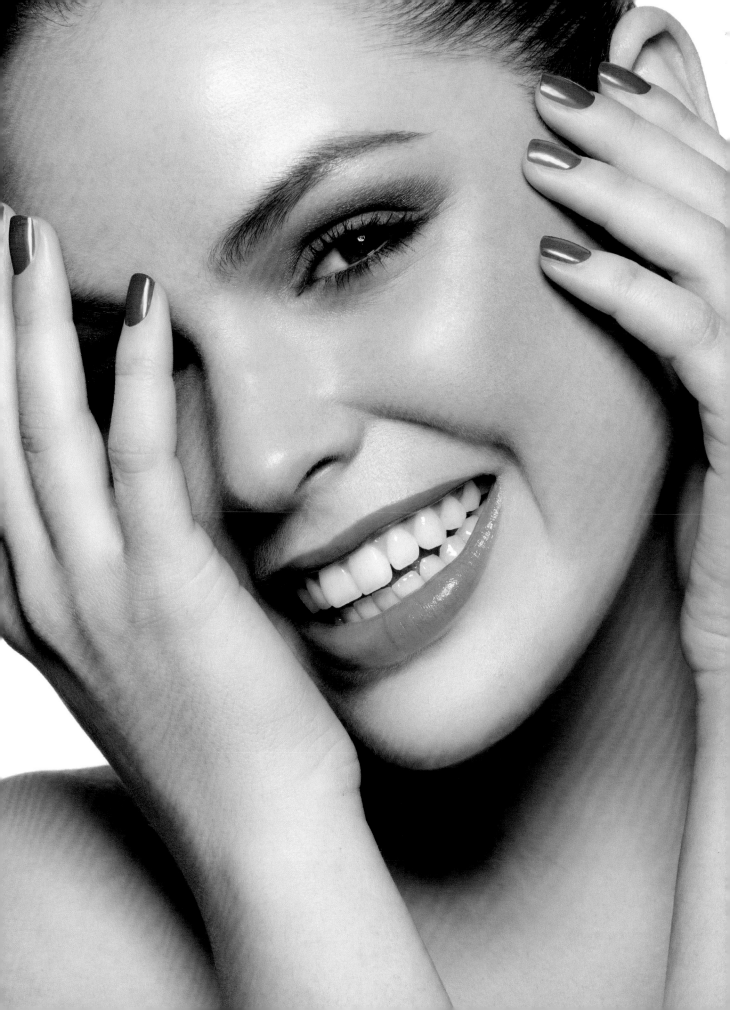

If you have oily skin...

Prepare the skin, don't just cover it. Create a canvas that will help to seal in the oils.

Use a gentle gel or foam cleanser formulated for oily skin (look for one containing Salicylic Acid) and avoid rich, creamy cleansers. Beware of using a harsh cleanser that will strip the sebum, the skin's natural oil, as your skin will overcompensate and produce more.

In spite of its oily surface, oily skin is often dehydrated and needs moisturizer to balance it and slow down its production of sebum.

Use a silicone-based primer under foundation to absorb any excess oil.

A powdered mineral foundation will help to keep oiliness at bay and will last longer on your skin. Make sure it has a matte finish, as any iridescence will look too shiny.

Without a good oil-absorbent base, wax- or oil-based cosmetics may slide, while powder eyeshadows and blushes can look patchy.

If you have dry skin...

Dry skin needs exfoliating at least three times a week to get rid of flakiness and dullness, and reveal the new, more radiant, smooth skin underneath. Removing the dry surface layer also makes it easier for moisturizer to penetrate.

Choose rich, creamy oil-based cleansers with a thick consistency. Don't overdry your face—keep it slightly damp, so that when you moisturize, you lock the moisture in.

Look for a moisturizer containing Hyaluronic Acid, as this is a great hydration booster.

Glycerine is another moisture-magnifying ingredient to look for.

Crème de la Mer is the most hydrating face cream there is—but it's a big outlay that perhaps isn't justifiable unless you have desert-dry skin.

Choose cream or liquid over powder foundations, and stay away from oil-free ones.

If you have sensitive skin...

Allergies, eczema, and rosacea are increasingly common, as sensitive skin can react to anything from chemicals to aromatherapy oils, leading to the release of neuroactive chemicals into the dermis causing burning and itching sensations.

Fragrance, or perfume, in cosmetics is one of the worst offenders, along with Sodium Laurel Sulphate, a foaming agent found in shower gels, shampoos, and toothpastes.

Chlorine in the water can aggravate skin conditions, so try using a special filter, such as a dechlorination bath ball or shower filter from the Sensitive Skincare Company.

Lack of sleep, pollution, a hectic lifestyle, and stress can all contribute to sensitive skin.

My first piece of advice is to consult a specialist for diagnosis and a recommended course of treatment.

Reduce the number of products you use and keep your regime as simple as possible.

Choose gentle products with no harsh chemicals and formulas designed to reduce redness.

Try to use only hypoallergenic products—Bare Minerals, Liz Earle, and Dove all do good ones.

KEY PRODUCTS TO PREP, PRIME, AND PROTECT

Always cleanse your face before you apply any products. This is especially important at the end of the day, when you need to get rid of all the pollution, dirt, and make-up that is clogging up your skin. Once you've cleansed, refresh the skin with cool water, and gently pat it dry with a clean towel.

SPF
UV radiation from the sun causes up to 90 percent of the skin's photoaging. Prevention is better than cure, as the old saying goes, so always apply SPF in the morning. Many daytime moisturizers and foundations contain SPF, but usually only up to Factor 15. I always wear SPF 50 in the summer and SPF 30 in the winter. Many skincare brands, such as Clarins, Origins, and Neutrogena, offer high SPF protection for the face combined with other skincare benefits.

MOISTURIZERS, EYE CREAMS, LIP BALM
Choose a formulation that is right for your skin (see page 156–9). Ideally use a day cream in the morning and a night cream, which tends to be richer, before bed. Use a prevention or correcting serum for your skin, if you need to (see Treatment, above right), then apply moisturizer to the face, neck, and décolletage and an eye cream around your eyes, patting them into the skin very gently.

A recent European study has shown that 52 percent of us describe our skin as sensitive.

TREATMENT
This includes serums, oils, creams (ones that have been medically prescribed to treat a particular condition), Retinol, eye gels, balms, and masks. What you choose will depend on your individual needs. Use them as directed—a mask is generally applied once a week, whereas serum or oil is usually used once or twice a day, under moisturizer.

PRIMER
Creating a smooth base, a primer holds make-up better than natural skin and gives a flawless, longer-lasting finish. Think of an artist preparing a canvas: primer is foundation's undercoat. Primers can be formulated to minimize pores, combat oiliness, hydrate, or illuminate, so choose one to suit your skin.

INSIDER SECRET
Moisturizer doesn't have to be expensive. Its main role is to create a barrier to keep moisture in: it's what you put inside your body that counts. There's no need to overcomplicate things—there are some very good inexpensive creams—I'm a big fan of Neutrogena and Olay.

FOUNDATION

Liquids, mousses, creams, sticks, mineral powders—there is a library of different formulas, colors, and finishes, so it really comes down to what you, as an individual, need and are looking for.

THE MAIN THINGS TO DECIDE ARE:

1 What level of coverage you require—high, medium, or sheer

2 What texture you prefer—matte, velvety, pearl, dewy, luminous

3 What is best for your skin type—oil-based or water-based

4 What shade(s) gives you a perfect match

Formulas & finishes

The foundation finish you choose is a personal choice. Some people prefer their skin matte, while others favor a more dewy look. A very dewy finish is great on the young, but as you grow older, a slightly more matte, softly luminous finish is the most flattering. Skin should never look oily or sweaty; you want the soft radiance of a child's skin—that youthful bloom—and a lot of that is down to good hydration. The two main types of foundation are oil- or water-based. Water-based foundations tend to give a more sheer, lightweight coverage, which looks really natural and is great for weekend use, teenagers, mature skin, or women who have good skin that just needs a bit of extra help. Water-based foundations are suitable for all, while oil-based foundations are more moisturizing for dry or dehydrated skin.

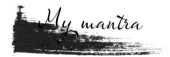

My mantra

Only apply foundation on areas of the face that really need it.

Mousse is very light and hydrating, giving a sheer coverage with a translucent finish that looks like your own skin. Mousse is good for most skin types, except extra-oily skin. A little goes a long way, so apply it sparingly.

1

Liquid foundation (1 and 2) is the most generic and is good for combination to dry skin; it is fairly hydrating and offers medium to full coverage.

2

Cream foundation (3) is rich and creamy, as its name suggests. It gives full, long-lasting coverage but is very hydrating, making it ideal for dry or mature skin.

3

Stick foundation provides heavier coverage, which is not so daylight-friendly but is good for blemished skin, evening use, or for photoshoots. Stick foundation is normally quite creamy, so you should think twice about using it if you have oily skin.

4

Powder foundation (4) feels light on the skin and buffs to a soft velvety finish. It normally contains minerals, so is very natural and a good choice for breakout-prone oily skin, as the sebum helps it absorb.

Color **Getting the color right is the absolute key—there is no greater make-up faux pas than when your face and neck are different colors. I'm a great believer in mixing shades of foundation to achieve a perfect match. No one has the same skin tone all year round, so I recommend having two similar shades of foundation—one slightly lighter and one slightly darker—and using them throughout the year to get the perfect color. You must have good natural light for this—if you get the color right in daylight, you'll look even more amazing in artificial light.**

PRO TRICK

Mix two shades of foundation together with a brush on the back of your hand, or on a plate, to achieve the perfect color match. Apply a little to your face, near your nose, and if it disappears into your skin and you can barely see it, then it's the right color. Use more or less of each shade as your skin changes color through the seasons.

tinted moisturizer

This is a relatively new product that women are still getting to grips with, but it is easy to use and can be very flattering. Treat it more like a moisturizer than a foundation and apply it all over your face using your fingers. Tinted moisturizer gives a very sheer, veil-like finish—more of a glow than coverage—which "lifts" the skin and makes it look hydrated and all-round better in a very natural, youthful way. Because it is so sheer, the colors are quite versatile and most skin tones can get away with using more than one shade. If you try one and it suits you, you will probably love it and never want to go back to using fuller coverage foundation.

Who can use it?

Tinted moisturizer won't cover blemishes and is sometimes not hydrating enough for very dry skin. It is ideal for anyone who has good skin that doesn't need camouflaging, but needs a little help to even out skin tone.

Some tinted moisturizers contain a higher SPF than foundation, so it is a good choice for summer.

It can be a good stepping-stone for fresh-faced teenagers getting into make-up.

Tinted moisturizer—especially one containing light-reflecting particles—is a great way of giving more mature skin a youthful glow. The pigment is not strong enough to settle in fine lines and creases.

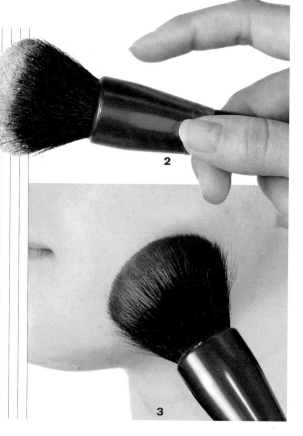

HOW TO APPLY FOUNDATION

I prefer applying nonpowder foundation with my fingers, as you can make sure you blend it really well, but you could use a foundation brush or sponge—whatever you find easier. Pat and press the product into the skin, rather than brushing or wiping it on and off in the same movement.

Apply powder foundation with a natural-bristle brush. Load the brush with product, swirl it around in the lid to work the powder into the bristles (1), tap it to remove the excess (2), and apply it to your face, starting at the outside and working inward (3). Buff it well with circular movements, really polishing your skin.

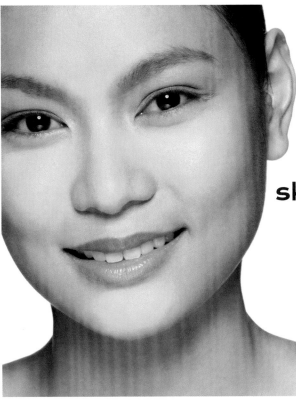

skin illuminators

Many primers and foundations contain pigments that reflect and bounce the light, giving skin the appearance of youthful radiance. Stand-alone skin illuminators, which have a brightening effect on dull skin, can be added to foundation or used on bare skin if you don't need coverage. This is a useful product for women later in life, because it restores the skin's natural glow.

color correctors and concealers

These products are used to disguise imperfections, blemishes, and skin discoloration—from birthmarks and redness to pimples and dark circles. Different color correctors are required to cover different types of blemishes. For example, a light yellow-based hue is needed to conceal dark purple/blue undereye circles, while a green tone is needed to neutralize redness—my Citrus Color Corrector (right) is a unique blend of both. An apricot color corrector (below right) brightens the skin and makes it look natural. I prefer moisturizing concealers with a creamy texture (below), which sink into the skin, rather than sit on the surface, and adhere well, so you can blend them properly without wiping them off. Apply concealer to bare skin or on top of foundation. You can blend colors to match your skin tone or layer them for greater coverage. Pat and push the product into the skin with a gentle twisting motion. Work it well into any fine lines and creases with a concealer brush and blend the edges outward so there are no hard lines. Set with fine translucent powder.

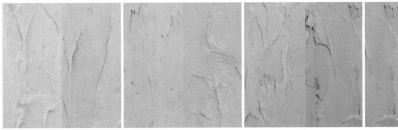

Fair **Light** **Medium** **Dark**

FACE SCULPTING

This is when you start playing with light and dark to contour your face and subtly change the features, enhancing, defining, lengthening, or shortening.

When done well, sculpting can transform a face. It can give women cheekbones they thought they never had, open up the eyes, soften strong jaws, and narrow wide noses (see pages 179 and 183). It's a technique that has been used in the theater for years, but there are ways of incorporating the principles into everyday make-up. The trick is to understand the planes of the face and learn where to apply the products.

GOLDEN RULE
Light brings features forward, dark pushes them back.

highlighting
Use highlighter to draw attention to certain areas that you want to "bring forward," but keep it away from crow's feet and fine lines, as you don't want to emphasize them. Apply it to the higher planes of the face that would naturally catch the light—especially cheekbones and browbones. The main thing is to be subtle. You don't want to strobe your skin so it looks like a glitterball, you want a soft luminosity as the light catches the pigments.

There isn't one universal highlighter for all skin tones, so choose one that suits yours. It mustn't look artificial, but should blend into your natural skin; if it's too light, it will look very silvery and obvious.

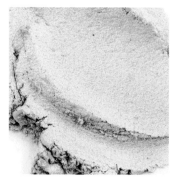

★ **Top tip** If your skin is oily, very dry, or sensitive, be careful with highlighter, because you don't want to emphasize problems.

If you have olive or deep skin, stay away from silver and white, and go for soft gold, rose gold, or copper—anything in that warm-toned spectrum, depending on how deep your skin tone is.

If you have very pale skin, use cream, eggshell, or vanilla, but don't be tempted to go too pale and, whatever you do, don't make it frosty—softly pearlized and luminous are what to aim for.

You can use cream or powder highlighter. Cream gives a more natural and youthful finish for daytime, especially if you are not wearing other powder products on your face. Powder highlighters are best used with heavier coverage foundation or when you are going to be under artificial lighting. Powder blends easiest on powder, so use a loose translucent powder under it to enable you to blend it subtly—you don't want any unevenness. Powder highlighter lasts longer, but it takes a little longer to apply.

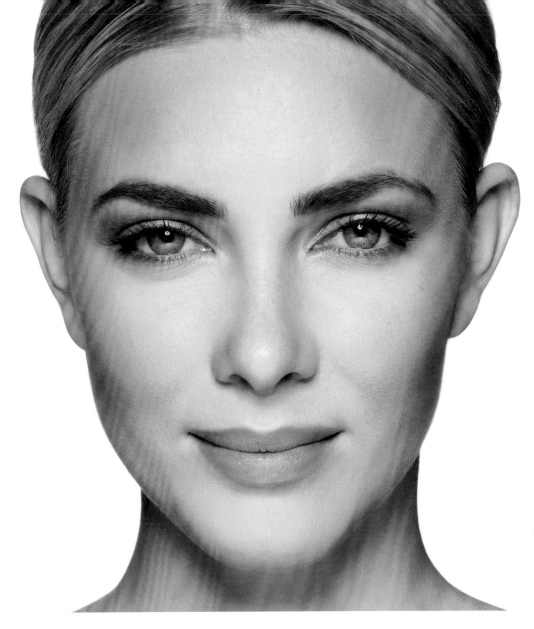

■ TOOL BOX

Colors that mimic shadows—matte, muddy, neutral, deeper tones—for contouring; and lighter products for highlighting and "lifting" areas of the face.

Contour Use a matte color one or two shades darker than your skin on areas you want to recede.

Highlight Blend a lighter product over the higher planes that would naturally catch the light.

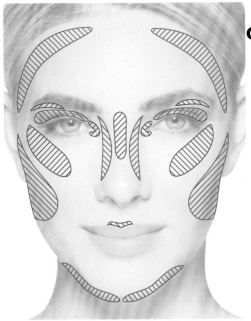

contour
Use matte, muddy colors for sculpting, to mimic natural shadows. Apply it where you want to take features or areas back, such as under the cheekbones to accentuate them by creating hollow cheeks, or in the crease of the eye socket to make eyes appear more open.

The color you choose should be one or two shades darker than your skin. I often use matte eyeshadows for contouring. Some people use lipsticks in brown tones, but make sure they are matte. You could also use cream or powder blushes in nude or skin-tone shades, or stick or cream foundations.

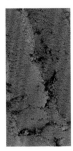

CREAM Apply cream blush with your finger or a synthetic brush for a light natural flush.

GET A HEALTHY GLOW

Blush warms up the skin and adds color to the cheeks, bringing a fresh, youthful glow to the face. Bronzer gives a healthy sunkissed look, as if you've just come back from vacation.

Blush adds the finishing touch to your look, and, best of all, it makes you look younger. Once we reach our mid-thirties, we begin to lose pigment in our skin, and that's when we need blush as a corrector instead of a fashion statement. You can apply it along the length of the cheekbones for a sophisticated look, or on the apples—the soft "pillows" when you smile—for a natural fresh-faced glow.

Colors range from brown tones—which include everything from deep reddish bronzes, to orange bronzes, right up to light brown and camel—to berry hues, pinks, corals, and peach/apricot tones.

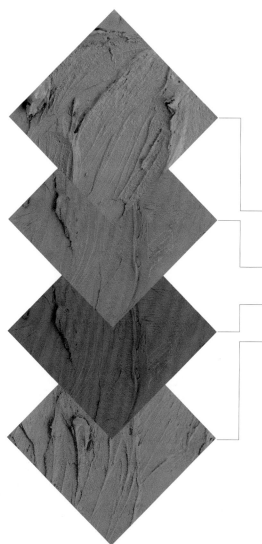

Peach/apricot tones are the most popular, the most versatile, and the most wearable colors, as they suit all skin tones.

Berry shades are more wintery, giving a stronger, more dramatic color.

Red and burgundy tones are very flattering on deep skins.

Pink shades can be quite difficult to wear, unless you have very pale skin. Dusky pinks are more wearable than bright bubblegum shades. (See pages 102–9).

PRO TRICK

Apply blush along the cheekbones or on the apples and blend it outward into the hairline. This gives a very natural look.

TINT Apply cheek tint
or stain with your
finger and blend it
quickly before it dries.
This gives long-lasting
sheer color that looks
very youthful.

POWDER
Use a natural-bristle blush brush to apply powder blush onto a powdered base, blending it well for an even, velvety finish.

GOLDEN RULES

You need a flawless base to wear blush well. A common mistake is to apply blush on skin that is blemished or uneven in tone—applying it on bare skin makes blemishes more obvious. To make blush as flattering as it can be, neutralize any natural redness on the face first.

Powder blush always blends best on a powdered base. Don't apply it to oily skin, as the pigments stick to the skin, making the color darker and harder to blend.

If you have good skin and only need a light foundation or tinted moisturizer, use gel, cream, or liquid stain on your cheeks.

For longer-lasting color, use a cream blush and then apply a little powdered blush over the top to set it.

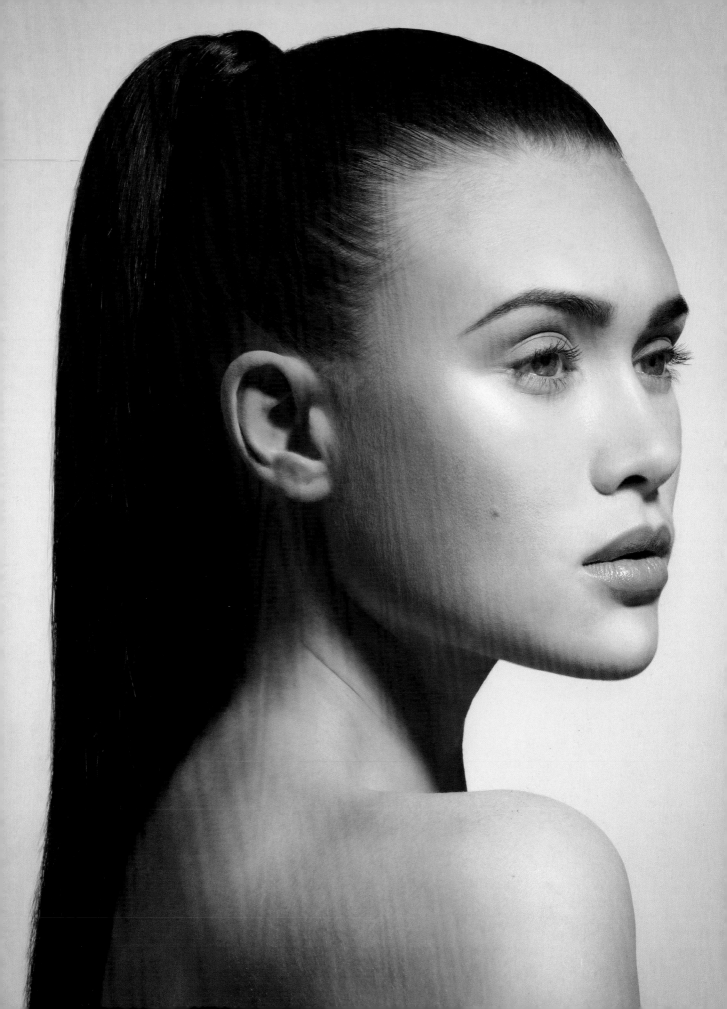

bronzer

Applied well, bronzer can be really flattering and convincing of a natural tan. You can use it to top up a real tan, too. Bronzer is most effective when applied over the side of the face and blended softly inward. Dust it where the sun naturally catches your face—on the T-zone (the nose, forehead, and chin) and cheekbones. Make sure you blend some over your neck, too, so that it matches your face. I prefer to use a smaller brush than a traditional bronzing brush, because it gives more control—the bigger the brush, the less control you have.

Much like blush, bronzer comes in different textures (gel, liquid, and powder), finishes (matte, luminous, and pearlized), and tones—from browns, through reds, to orange, peach, and gold. I favor powder bronzer with a soft pearl finish.

It is essential to use the right shade, taking into account the time of year. Prism or streaked bronzers are made up of lots of colors, so you can tailor-make the right shade for you. One bronzer in my range is a trio of shades, so you can go slightly paler in the winter and slightly darker in the summer, subtly lifting the skin without it looking artificial.

PRO TRICK

Blend bronzer from the hairline, gradually working it into the face so the effect is softer there.

Apply bronzer where indicated by the shading, blending it well and working from the outside in.

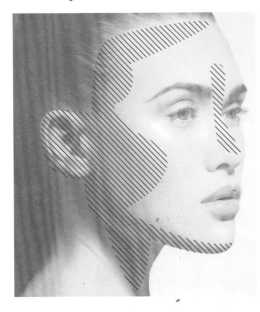

GOLDEN RULES

\# It is difficult to use bronzer on pale skin, because the contrast is too great. It is better to use an apricot or pinky peach blush and then just dust a light sprinkling of bronzer on top to warm it up. You could also warm up your skin with foundation or tinted moisturizer before application. If you have really milky skin, stay away from bronzer.

\# Pearly textures can look lovely, but only in the summer.

\# Be precise in your application—a common mistake is to use a brush that is way too big for the face. This gives no control and results in the dreaded all-over-orange effect.

\# Don't draw a cross down and across your face and then sweep the brush round and round—this gives you that classic lollipop head.

\# Don't go more than two shades darker than your skin tone.

CREATING PERFECT SKIN THE PRO WAY

When I'm making someone up, whether it's for an event, a photoshoot, or TV, the first thing I always do is feel their skin. Most people have dehydrated skin, especially around the nose and on the cheeks. If the skin feels like sandpaper, I cleanse it, then hydrate it with a rich, nourishing cream, which I leave to absorb for 10–15 minutes before reapplying if necessary. Then I look to see whether they have clear skin or whether there are blemishes and areas that need covering.

The level of cover depends on the job. If it's a photoshoot or TV appearance I apply more coverage, but if it's a wedding or an event I put on less and use lighter formulations.

For photoshoots and TV the finish has to be completely flawless and mattified—any oil on the skin under bright lights turns the face into a disco ball. I might use cream blush for the intensity of color, but I'd always set it with powder.

For a wedding the focus is on creating the most natural, perfect skin, which needs to look good in daylight—the most unforgiving light. I only cover areas that need it, evening out the skin tone with concealer, as necessary, and then using a light foundation with slight luminosity to make the skin look healthy and alive. For the cheeks, I'd use cream, gel, or liquid stain, which look very natural in daylight.

CHECKLIST: KEY PRODUCTS

These are what I consider to be the essential products to have in your beauty kit. How many of them you choose to buy is entirely up to you—you may use some every day and others only on special occasions. My advice is to use everything in the first category on a regular basis. If you invest in your skin long-term, you will need fewer products to correct and enhance.

Skincare

Cleanser
Treatment serum/oil
SPF
Moisturizer—for day, night, eyes, and lips

Complexion perfectors

Primer
Foundation (or tinted moisturizer)
Color corrector
Concealer
Skin illuminator
Powder/setting spray

Enhancers

Eyeshadows
Eyeliners
Mascara
Brow kit (tweezers, brow brush, powder, or pencil)
Blush
Bronzer
Highlighter
Lipsticks
Gloss

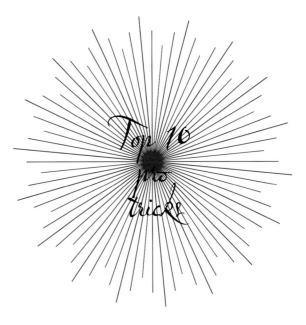

Top 10 Make-up tricks

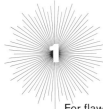

1

For flawless skin, prep, prime, and protect before adding color—cleanse, apply SPF, then use a primer to provide a smooth, long-lasting base.

2

Don't cover good skin—only apply color correctors, concealer, and foundation where you need them.

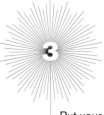

3

Put your make-up on in good natural light, using a big mirror. Don't use a magnifying mirror—it will only make you depressed.

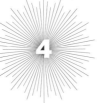

4

Tame your brows—pluck, thread, wax, whichever you prefer. Grooming your brows opens up your eyes and makes a huge difference to your whole face (see pages 66–9).

5

If you've got problem skin, see a specialist. Don't try to self-diagnose. You will save yourself a lot of time, money, and angst in the long run.

6

A spot can completely ruin your day if you let it. Don't let it.

7

It's not about what you put on your skin, it's about what you put in your body. Bad skin starts from within (see pages 162–7).

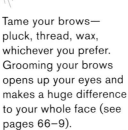

8

Don't let your eye make-up fight with your lipstick. If you're going for strong eyes, let them be the focus and keep your lips natural. If you're going for a bold mouth, keep your eyes more subtle.

9

Always cleanse and moisturize, morning and night. I say "always," but of course there will be times when you let this slip—just don't make it a regular thing. And remember, you don't need to spend a fortune on cleanser and moisturizer. The key is to get the dirt and make-up off and lock the moisture in.

10

Sleep. This is important, especially as you get older. A good night's rest does wonders for your face—and your mood, which only makes you look better than ever.

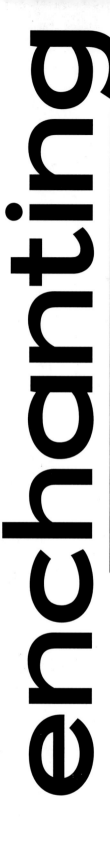

enchanting

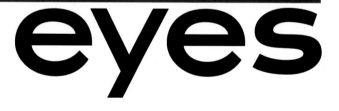

Eye make-up can be used in so many different ways to define and enhance your eyes. All it takes is a little product knowledge and some simple techniques to create an almost infinite number of looks, from classic and pretty, to bold and edgy, to dramatic and theatrical.

eyes

Making up your eyes is not difficult once you have learned a few basic principles and skills. Eyeliner, eyeshadow, and mascara are perhaps the most versatile of all make-up—available in myriad colors and textures that give you the opportunity to play around and experiment with different effects to see what suits you. The combination of products you use, how much you apply, and where and how you apply them will result in very different finished looks.

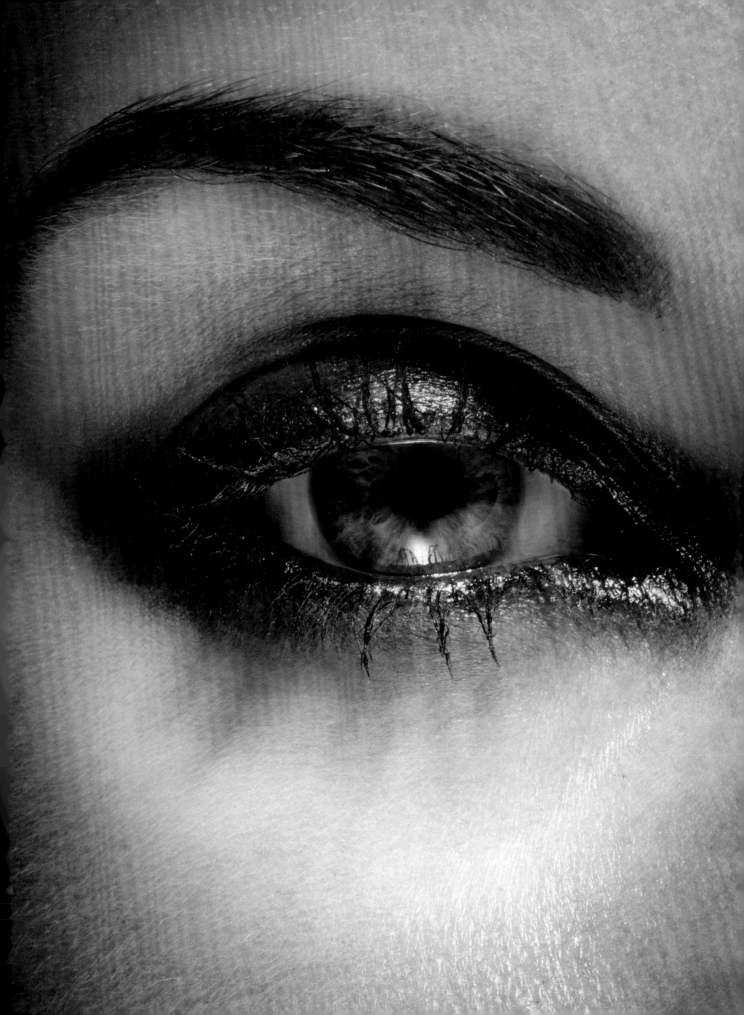

EYE

How to apply make-up to flatter different eye shapes is one of the topics I am asked about most.

SHAPE

My view is that make-up should always be used to enhance your features to best effect, and there are a few simple principles to bear in mind when making up your eyes, taking into account their shape, how they are set in your face, and the size of your eyelids.

GOLDEN RULE

Highlighting an area with a light color or shimmery texture will make it stand out (indicated by the blue dots on the diagrams); a dark color or matte texture will deepen the area or make it recede (indicated by the red shading on the diagrams).

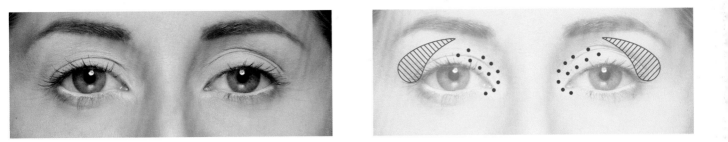

close-set eyes

If the space between your eyes is less than the width of one eye, you have close-set eyes. To create the illusion that the eyes are farther apart, emphasize the outer part of the eyes with darker eyeshadows (see the red shaded area, above right) and use a paler color on the inner part (see the blue dotted area).

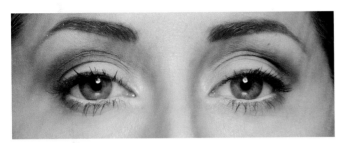

Classic day look

1 After priming the eyes (see page 44), brush neutral bone-colored powder eyeshadow over the whole eyelid, from the lash line up to the browbone.

2 Apply brown pencil eyeliner along the roots of the upper lashes for definition, starting about a third of the way along from the inner corners.

3 Brush a darker toning eyeshadow over the eyeliner, taking it onto the roots of the lower lashes at the outer corners. Then blend it into the socket crease at the outer part of the eyes.

4 Curl the lashes and apply lengthening mascara, focusing on the outer lashes.

Nighttime transformation

1 Use a deep brown eyeshadow to contour the sockets, blending it out for a winged effect.

2 Apply gel eyeliner to the upper lash lines, bringing it beyond the corner of the eyes and creating a subtle flick to elongate and lift the outer corners.

3 Blend the eyeshadow along the roots of the lower lashes to make the eyes look bigger.

4 Apply another coat of lengthening mascara to the top lashes and the outer corner of the bottom lashes. Then apply corner lashes.

PRO TRICKS

Pale eyeshadow on the inner three-quarters of your lids gives the impression of more space between the eyes.

Emphasize the outer third of your lids with a darker color and blend it out to elongate the eyes.

Highlight under the browbones and on the tear ducts.

Keep eyeliner to the outer corners and smudge it inward. Draw a fine line that takes up less lid space.

Create the illusion of larger eyes by using nude or flesh-colored eyeliner on the inner rims.

A touch of brighter eyeshadow right in the middle of the eyelids will magnify your eyes.

Use a taupe eyeshadow underneath the bottom lashes to create the effect of slightly larger eyes.

Emphasize the outer lashes with more mascara.

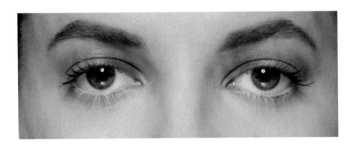
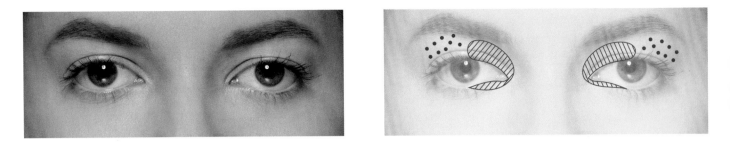

wide-set eyes
If the space between your eyes is greater than the width of one eye, you have wide-set eyes. To make the eyes seem closer together, draw the focus inward by emphasizing the inner half of the eyes with deeper colors (see the red shaded area, above right) and keeping lighter colors to the outer half of the eyes (see the blue dotted area).

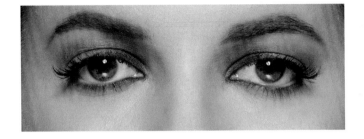

Classic day look

1. Begin by priming the eyes to create a neutral base (see page 44), then bring the focus inward by applying a soft mocha eyeshadow to the inner third of the eyes and blending it from the lash line up onto the lid.
2. Apply a toning eyeshadow in a lighter color to the outer part of the lash line, blending it up above the socket crease but not outward.
3. Use a blending brush to ensure there are no hard edges where the two colors meet.
4. Curl the lashes and apply a coat of mascara.

Nighttime transformation

1. Deepen the intensity of color at the inner corners, working it into the socket crease.
2. Take the deeper color onto the lower lash line at the inner corners, blending it softly toward the outer corners.
3. Touch up the caramel eyeshadow on the outer part of the lid, blending it upward and inward.
4. Apply another coat of mascara to the top and bottom lashes.

PRO TRICKS

You can use eyeliner all around the eyes, even on the inner rims, so a smoky eye will work well on you (see pages 70–5).

Avoid a cat's-eye shape or a flick at the outer corners, as they will make your eyes seem more wide-set.

Apply a dark, matte eyeshadow at the inner corners and blend it to about one-third of the way across the eyelids.

Blend a lighter shade toward the outer corners, but don't take it beyond the eyes.

Emphasize the sockets, concentrating on the inner half of the eyes and blending it to fade toward the outer corners.

Concentrate mascara application on the inner lashes.

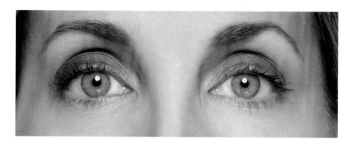
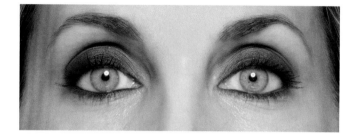

prominent eyes

If your eyes protrude from your face, you have prominent eyes. Use dark colors and matte textures on the upper and lower lids to push the eyes back (see the red shaded area, above right), and highlight the browbones to bring them forward (see the blue dotted areas). Avoid light-reflecting eyeshadows, which will bring the lids farther forward.

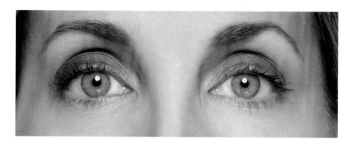

Classic day look

1. Prime the eyes (see page 44) and then apply a soft pearl taupe eyeshadow over the mobile lid, focusing on the outer half of the eye.
2. Blend a little bone-colored eyeshadow onto the outer part of the browbone to highlight it.
3. Curl the lashes and apply one coat of mascara.

Nighttime transformation

1. Accentuate the upper and lower lash lines by working black pencil eyeliner into the roots of the lashes.
2. Apply dark gray powder eyeshadow over the pencil eyeliner and blend it up onto the lid for a soft finish.
3. Blend more of the taupe eyeshadow into the socket, working the colors together well.
4. Apply another coat of mascara to the lashes.

PRO TRICKS

- # Focus on matte, velvety, or soft pearl textures on the lids, but avoid anything with too much shimmer.
- # Use camels, taupes, and darker shades, not bright colors that will draw attention to the lids.
- # Don't emphasize the sockets, and focus on contouring.

- # Apply the same color eyeshadow along the bottom lash lines, especially at the outer corners, blending it softly inward. This will set the entire eye area slightly back.
- # If you wear eyeliner, keep it soft and blend it up into the eyeshadow, so there are no hard lines along the roots of the lashes.

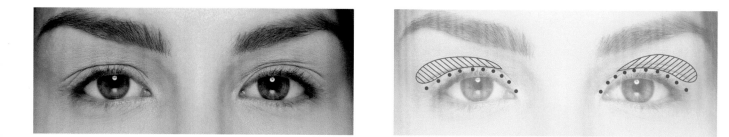

deep-set eyes
If your eyes are sunk into the sockets, or if your lids are heavy with prominent browbones, you have deep-set eyes. Bring the eyes forward, using lighter colors to lessen the shadows on the inside corners and upper lash lines (see the blue dotted area, above right), and make the browbones recede with deeper colors (see the red shaded area).

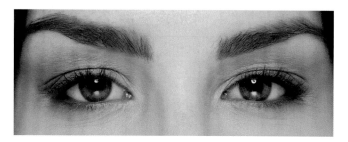

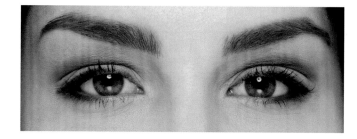

Classic day look

1 Prime the eyes (see page 44) and then apply a natural beige powder eyeshadow as a light colorwash all over the lids, blending it from the lash lines to the browbones.

2 Apply a darker contour shade along the socket creases, stopping just above the inner edge of the iris and blending well.

3 Define and highlight the upper lash line with purple eyeshadow.

4 Blend the same color along the lower lash line at the outer corners to balance the eyes.

5 Curl the lashes to open up the eyes and apply a coat of lengthening mascara.

Nighttime transformation

1 Use a taupe brown eyeshadow to contour the sockets, blending it outward and upward to make the eyes appear wider.

2 Blend a shimmery champagne eyeshadow on the inner corners of the eyes and over the mobile lids to bring them forward.

3 Apply brown pencil eyeliner along the upper lash lines and outer corners of the lower lash lines.

4 Define the lower lash lines with taupe brown eyeshadow at the roots of the lashes.

5 Apply another coat of lengthening mascara to the upper lashes and a very light coat to the lower lashes.

PRO TRICKS

\# Apply light shimmery eyeshadow on the eyelids up to the sockets to bring the lids forward.

\# Blend an eyeshadow one shade darker than your skin tone into the sockets, focusing on the outer corners, to give depth and definition.

\# Draw eyeliner along the upper lash lines to just past the outer corner, keeping it fine so as not to lose lid space. You could also try tightlining (see page 52).

\# Line the lower lashes from the outer corners inward, to just below the pupil, and smudge gently.

\# Curl the lashes to open up the eyes, then apply lots of volumizing mascara on the top lashes only.

\# If your lids are hooded, blend a darker shade from the lash lines to the sockets to push them back. Line both lash lines, focusing on elongating the eyes—feline shapes and flicks work well.

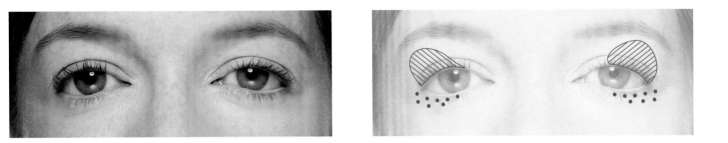

downward-sloping eyes
If your eyes tilt down at the outer corners, they can make you look sad and tired. Focus on bringing the outer corners of the eyes up with deeper colors (see the red shaded area, above right)—a flick would work well. Use a pale color under the outer corner of the eyes to create "lift" (see the blue dotted area).

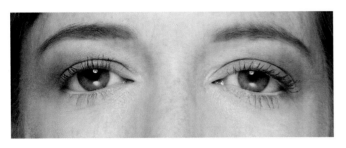

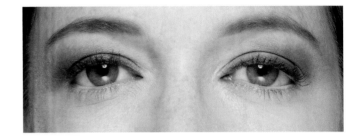

Classic day look

1 Prime the eyes (see page 44) and then apply a wash of neutral warm peachy beige eyeshadow over the mobile lids.

2 Blend a deeper toning shade onto the outer part of the eyes, from the lash line to the socket crease. Soften the edges and focus on creating lift by blending the color up above the crease.

3 Apply a pale skin-tone eyeshadow under the outer part of the lower lashes to brighten and lift the downward-sloping corners.

4 Curl the lashes to open up the eyes and apply lengthening mascara.

Nighttime transformation

1 Give the eyes greater definition by working a deeper brown eyeshadow along the upper lash lines, right at the roots of the lashes, but stop just before you reach the outer corners.

2 Take the darker shade up from the lash lines and into the sockets above the outer third of the eye, blending it well.

3 Apply another coat of mascara to the upper lashes, lifting them at the outer corners.

PRO TRICKS

When you use eyeliner, draw it from the center of the upper lash line outward, but instead of following the natural shape of the eye as it slopes down, concentrate on creating lift.

If you use eyeliner on the lower lash lines, stop just in from the outer corners and smudge it for a soft effect.

Apply a pale or mid-color eyeshadow over the whole lid, then blend a darker shade into the socket, but start lifting it a fraction in from the outer corners and blend it outward and upward.

Curl the lashes well to help open up the eyes.

EYESHADOW / APPLICATION

There are lots of ways to apply eyeshadow, from a simple colorwash to a contoured smoky eye. Once you have mastered the basic three-step technique, you will be able to try your hand at any look.

This is the failsafe way to apply any color of eyeshadow—it works just as well for nude tones as for gray, purple, or green shades. You can just use step 1, stop at step 2, or take it all the way to step 3, depending on the level of definition that you want to achieve.

1 Apply a light wash of the palest color from the lash line to the browbone.

2 Take the mid-tone and lightly blend it into the eye socket. Add a small amount along the bottom lash line using a pencil-shaped brush.

3 Smudge the darkest color along the upper lash line, concentrating on the outer corner. Create a C-shape at the outer corner, curving round from the lash line and into the socket.

HOW TO PREP YOUR EYES

Prep your eyes first to ensure the eyeshadow color is true and lasts longer. Use an eye primer (Nars makes a good one) or a dab of foundation or creamy concealer to neutralize any redness on the eyelids or dark shadows under the eyes. Then brush the eyelids with a little translucent powder to absorb moisture and create a smooth base.

Use a soft, fluffy eye brush and a windshield-wiper motion to blend, blend, blend, working over any line where there is a change of color.

Top tip When it comes to make-up beneath the eye—on or just under the lower lash line—use the make-up above the eye as a guide: you never want more make-up below the eye than above it. The idea is to create a lifting effect, so avoid anything that draws the focus downward.

EYE MAP

1 Browbone
2 Socket crease
3 Mobile lid
4 Lash line
5 Tear ducts
6 Waterline/inner rim
7 Lower lash line
8 Line of elevation

PRO TRICK

Work out your line of elevation. Take a make-up brush or pencil and hold it from the outer corner of your eyebrow to the outer corner of the bottom of your nose. Where the brush crosses your eye area is the line below which you shouldn't apply any make-up. Keep all your eye make-up within this line and don't take it below: this gives the effect of a mini eyelift and keeps your eyes looking clean and bright.

EYESHADOW

Available in a rainbow of colors to suit every skin tone and to make every eye color "pop," eyeshadows are either powder or cream in texture, with finishes ranging from matte and velvety to pearl, metallic, and gloss.

TEXTURES, FINISHES, AND COLORS

powder

Pressed-powder eyeshadows are the staples and are perfect for everyday. Loose eyeshadows are best for highlighting or accessorizing your look with a dab at the inner corners of your eyes. They come in a good range of colors and are normally very high in pigment, so are great for creating a pop of color. Loose shadow works really well layered with cream shadow and pressed into it. It is easy to blend but can be very messy to apply.

Finishes

Pearl eyeshadows are the easiest to blend and have a shimmery light-reflecting effect. They are the most wearable, versatile, and flattering eyeshadows.

Metallic eyeshadows give an eye-catching finish and you can use them to create dramatic, high-fashion or party looks.

Matte eyeshadows are great for adding extra shading and definition. They can also be used wet to line the eyes.

☐ TOOL BOX

Cream powders are best applied with a wand or synthetic brush, which won't absorb the product, while powder shadows should be blended with soft natural-bristle brushes, such as squirrel, goat, pony, or sable. Use a flat brush to apply the shadow, pressing it into the skin, and then smudge and blend it well with a blending brush.

cream

Eye crayons, liquid eyeshadows, and cream eyeshadows that come in palette form are all types of cream. Cream shadows often have a metallic or pearl finish to give a wet look; they tend to crease very quickly and aren't ideal for long wear. Eye crayons and liquid shadows that come in a mascara-like tube tend to be longer lasting and less likely to crease. I prefer to layer cream shadows under powder textures, which gives them greater staying power and intensity of color.

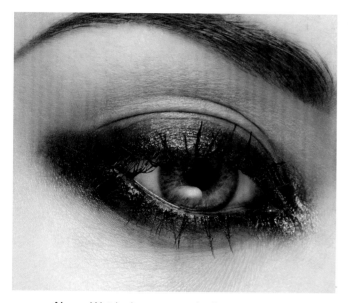

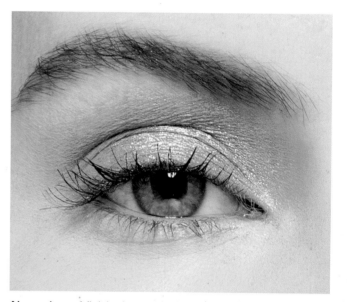

Above Wet-look cream eyeshadow can be used for many high-fashion looks. **Below** A metallic finish creates a striking effect and gold is flattering on warm skin.

Above A pearl finish gives a soft light-reflecting effect that is highly flattering. **Below** Matte eyeshadow is best for creating depth, shading, and definition.

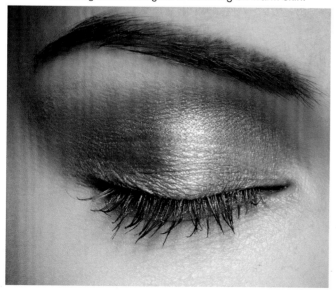

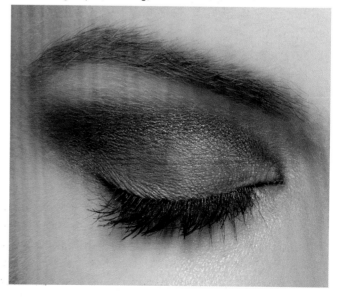

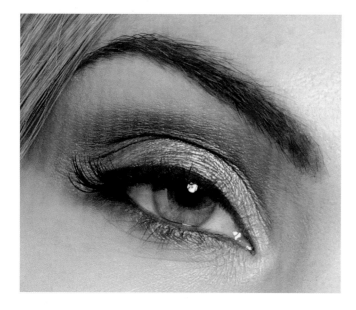

Above Eyeshadows in colors that blend with the skin tone give subtle definition. **Below** A light colorwash of soft beige-gold creates the perfect nude eye.

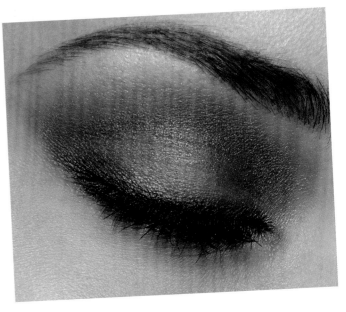

Above Slate-gray powder eyeshadow with a soft pearl finish is flattering on cool skin tones. **Below** Green eyeshadow intensifies the color of green eyes.

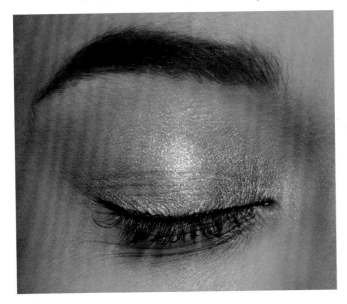

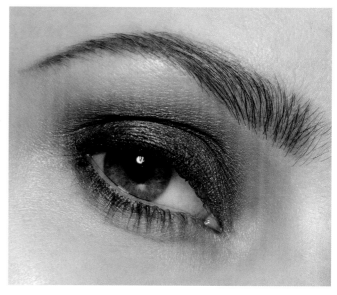

colors Take into account your skin tone and the
color of your iris when you are choosing eyeshadows. If you have warm skin (with yellow or orange undertones), warm colors with an orange or gold base will be most flattering; if you have cool skin (with pink or red undertones), cooler colors with a blue or silvery base and pink-based warmer colors will suit you best.

When it comes to eye color, take your cue from a 12-color artist's wheel. Any three colors adjacent to each other on the wheel are "related." Choose a palette of related colors to intensify your eye color. "Complementary" colors are those that are directly opposite each other on the wheel and these, or tones of these, will make your eye color pop.

PRO TRICK
Loose glitter is a fun way to create easy, instant party looks. Dust it over powder eyeshadows or press it into cream eyeshadows.

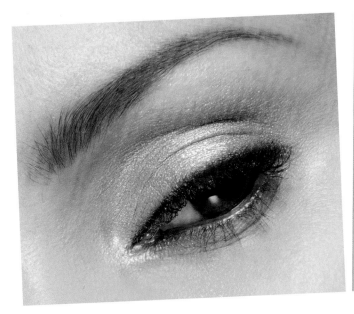

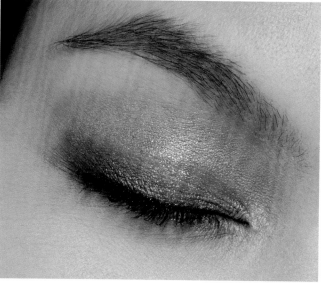

Above Black eyeliner is essential to frame the silver pigment blended onto cream eyeshadow. **Below** A dramatic look is achieved with a bright pink colorwash.

Above The dark bronze defining the lash line is blended out into a softer shade. **Below** Purple flatters most eye colors and can be used for subtle or bold effects.

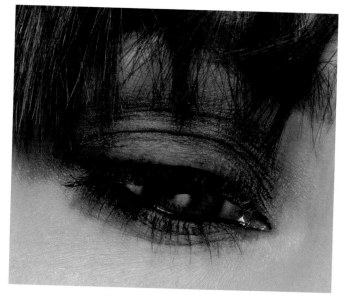

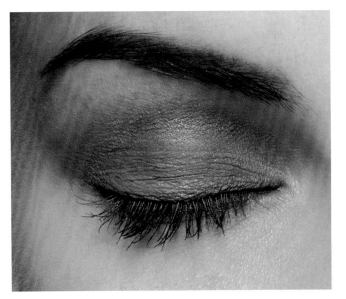

HELPFUL HINT

Buy the best-quality eyeshadow you can. There are exceptions but, as a rule, buying cheaper eyeshadows is a false economy, because the pigment is often not as strong so you have to use more. Test the eyeshadow before you buy by putting a dab of the color on the back of your hand—this will show you the texture, the finish, and the payoff (how strong the color is). It is all to do with the consistency of the powder—the finer it is, the better it will blend; if the particles are too big, it won't blend and sit on the skin well. Guerlain and Christian Dior make some of the best high-end eyeshadows, while ELF offers good economy options.

COLORS TO MAKE YOUR EYES POP

Blue eyes Orange tones, such as golden brown, copper, terracotta, peach

Green eyes Red tones, such as pink, violet, burgundy, plum

Brown eyes Brown doesn't have a complementary color, but purples and greens look great with brown eyes

Hazel eyes Blue, violet, purple, and red tones complement the orange and green flecks in hazel eyes

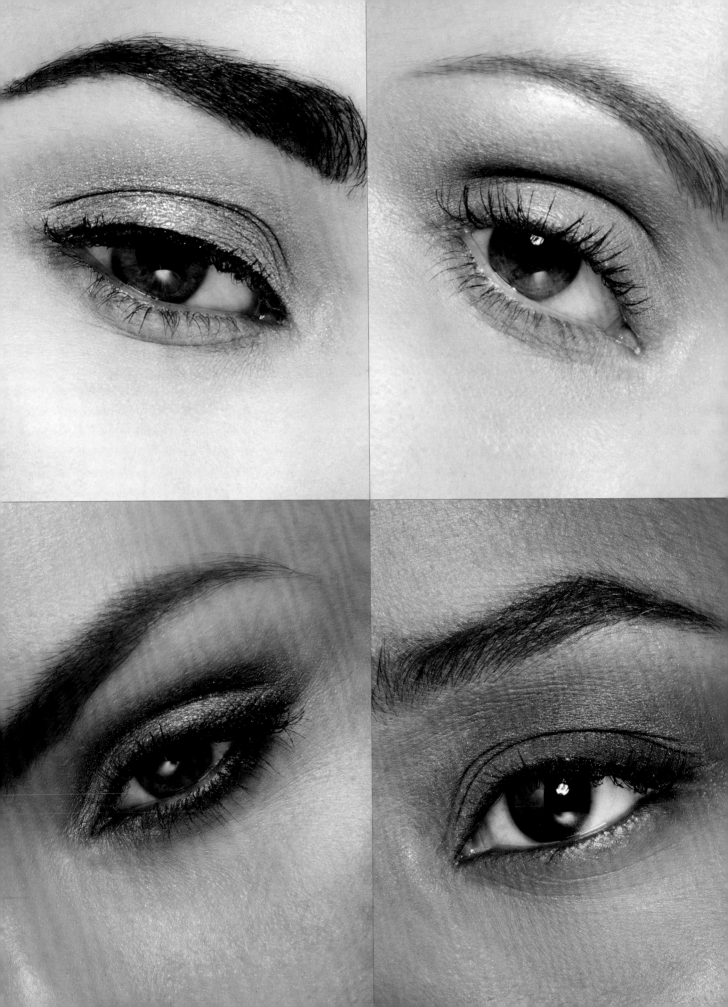

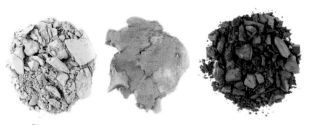

Perfect eyeshadow for porcelain skin

Cool colors with silver and blue undertones suit porcelain skin, whereas yellow, gold, or orange undertones clash. Grays and silvery or blue-based pinks look great. Ivory is a better choice of nude than the warmer, wheaty shades. Silver, which can be difficult to wear, flatters cool skin tones and intensifies blue and green eyes, which often go hand in hand with a porcelain complexion.

Silver powder was pressed on top of silver cream, which holds the pigment and intensifies the color. Light bone-colored eyeshadow under the browbones provides subtle highlighting. The eyes are framed by strong brows and thin liquid eyeliner along the upper lash lines. The lashes need to be dark and defined to balance the pale eyeshadow.

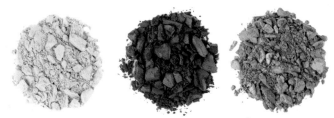

Perfect eyeshadow for fair skin

Fair skin has warmer undertones and often goes with brown or hazel eyes, so you can play with more colors and make the transition into warmer shades. Warm browns, taupes, and soft golds work well, but don't go all the way to orange. You can still use silvery highlighter and cooler shades to tone down anything that is too warm for your coloring. You can also mix camels and silvers, and wear greens, blues, and cooler lilacs and purples.

This eye illustrates how someone with fair skin can wear cool and warm tones together without them clashing. The silvery highlight under the brow works well with the taupe on the lid and the deeper brown defining the socket crease.

Perfect eyeshadow for olive skin

Colors with gold and orange undertones are the most flattering for olive skin, which has a rich warm tone and often goes with brown eyes. You can wear greens and red-based purples, but go for the deep shades, such as olive, eggplant, and plum, and mix them with gold highlights.

I wanted to show how fabulous a strong orange-bronze can look with olive skin and brown eyes—it's a classic combination. Earth-brown pencil eyeliner was worked into the roots of the lashes and along the upper and lower lash lines, and blended out into a subtle flick to elongate the eye. The rich bronze eyeshadow has a high pearl finish that catches the light.

Perfect eyeshadow for deep skin

Generally, deep skin can carry off more dramatic eyeshadows than paler skin tones. The darker your skin, the more blue its undertone, so cool colors will suit you best; the lighter your skin, the more green or yellow its undertone, so warm hues will be more flattering. Experiment—there is an array of colors that suit you.

This skin tone has a lovely rich warmth to it with deep olive undertones and looks fabulous with the red-based purply brown eyeshadow that is just a couple of shades darker than the skin. The soft pearl finish and gold highlights soften the color and make it highly flattering.

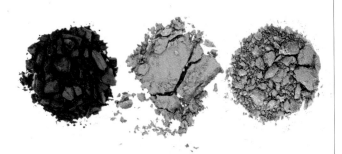

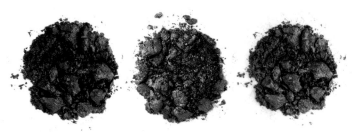

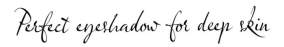

EYELINER

There are many ways to line the eyes using pencil, liquid, gel, or powder eyeliner. You can create everything from a fine, soft line for natural-looking definition, to statement feline shapes that are pure drama.

TIGHTLINING This is when eyeliner is applied on the inner rim of the eye, at the very roots of the lashes, to subtly define the eye without taking up any lid space. Using a gel or pencil eyeliner, look straight into a mirror, lift up your upper lashes, and apply the eyeliner along the inner rim.

Pencil eyeliner

Pencil is the most easy-to-use and versatile eyeliner, allowing you to create a sexy smudged eye or a sharp flick. Look for a creamy pencil that is soft to go on and easy to blend, but with a long-lasting, water-resistant finish.

Liquid liner

This is probably the most difficult eyeliner to apply, but practice makes perfect. Keep your hand steady by resting your elbow on a table as you work.

Gel eyeliner

I love gel eyeliner: you can achieve the same effects as with liquid liner, but it is easier to apply and lasts longer. You can also press powder eyeshadow into gel liner, making it really versatile (this is a great way to create a smoky eye). Available in many colors, gel liner comes in a pot and has a texture similar to shoe polish. Apply it with a fine-tipped brush, building up the color in increments.

Powder

You can use most eyeshadows as eyeliners, applying them wet or dry using a fine-tipped brush to create the desired shape. Powder eyeliner offers a wide choice of colors, is easy to blend, and creates a softer finish.

Glitter eyeliner

A fun accessory that is great for party looks, glitter eyeliner has the consistency of regular gel eyeliner and is an easy way to glam up your lash line with a dash of glitter.

eyeliner effects

I wanted to demonstrate how the color and texture of the eyeliner you use influences the end result as much as how you apply it. Here, the same eye has been made up using black and brown pencil eyeliner (below left) and black gel liner (opposite) to create very different effects.

1

2

3

Pencil eyeliner

Black pencil (1) is a good choice for the evening or for dramatic looks, as it helps to frame the eyes and pop eyeshadow colors, especially the cooler tones. Its application needs to be really precise, as any imperfections or mistakes will be emphasized. Black goes with warm and cool colors, and stands out well on darker skin tones.

Brown pencil (2 and 3) gives a softer, more wearable look than harsher black, making it perfect for daytime or older women—I always advise ladies to stick to brown eyeliner once they are in their late forties. There are lots of shades, from warm caramel to deep earthy brown. Wear brown liner with warm hues of eyeshadow, as it doesn't work so well with cool colors.

Pencil liner can be applied to the top lash line only (2), or you can work it under the lashes at the outer corner and blend it to about a third of the way along the lower lash line, too (3).

TOP TIPS FOR APPLYING EYELINER

\# When applying liquid liner, draw out the shape in pencil first before going over it with the liquid.

\# Apply liquid and gel liner sparingly using a thin, supple brush, building it up gradually—this is the best way to prevent smearing and running.

\# Clean up any mistakes using a Q-tip dipped in concealer; then dip the other end into translucent powder and apply it over the same area to set it.

\# Lining the inner rim of the eye with a creamy white or flesh-colored pencil is a great way to open up the eyes.

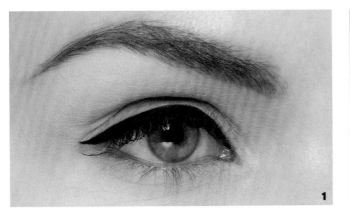

1

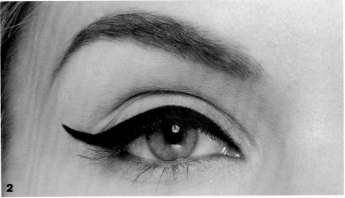

2

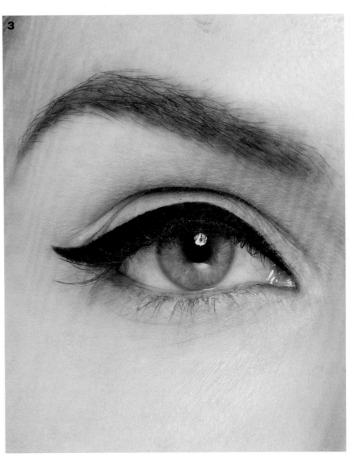

3

Gel or liquid liner flicks

A classic flick (1) is a great way to extend your natural eye, making it more feline and elongated in shape. Don't follow the curve of the lash line at the outer corner, as that will pull your eyes downward and make them look droopy. Instead, bring the liner out horizontally, making sure it tails off just above the outer corner of the eyes.

The elongated flick (3) first became fashionable in the 1950s and is still a popular evening look. Follow the shape of the eye from the inner corner of the upper lash line to just before the outer corner and then flick the tail upward, which gives the illusion of lifting the eye up at the outer corners. This is a difficult look to achieve if you have deep-set or hooded eyes, as you need to be able to see the eyelid. The trick is to get the right shape: make sure the line tapers toward the inner corner of the eye, is at its thickest in the middle and then begins to slim out two-thirds of the way along with an upward flick just above the outer corner.

The party flick (2) is a more extreme version of the elongated flick and creates a real statement. Think modern-day Cleopatra.

TOP TIPS FOR CREATING A FLICK

\# Pros can draw a flick in one fluid line but little movements are easier, so start by building up the line gradually so that if you make a mistake it will be easier to resolve.

\# Look straight into a mirror with your chin up, so that you can really see the shape of your eye.

\# If you are not confident about where the line should go, draw the flick lightly in pencil first and then go over it with the liquid or gel liner.

LUSH LASHES

Eye make-up never really looks right until the mascara is on. It gives the finishing touch to any eye look and completely changes the face—it's the icing on the cake.

TOP TIPS

Mascara should be replaced every few months because of the risk of a build-up of bacteria. When you buy a new mascara smell it, and as soon as it smells different, throw it away.

Make sure you close your mascara tightly so that it doesn't dry out.

Pumping the wand doesn't ensure even distribution but forces air into the tube, which dries out the product.

Mascara is most women's number-one desert-island make-up essential and it's where cosmetics manufacturers make most of their money. Consequently, a lot of research goes into creating ever-improving formulations. There is an overwhelming choice on the market, claiming to lengthen, curl, volumize, separate, and it can be really baffling to know which to choose—even within an individual brand there can be a choice of as many as eight different mascaras. Two of my favorites are Benefit's They're Real! and L'Oréal's False Lash Telescopic Mascara.

HOW TO CURL YOUR LASHES

Always curl the lashes before you apply mascara, as it really helps to open and lift the eyes. To create a natural swoop of lash, rather than a harsh right-angle bend, crimp the lashes as close as you can to the roots, then halfway along, and lastly right at the ends. You can squeeze the curlers quite hard but don't pull: squeeze, count to three, open, and release. Never curl your lashes after applying mascara, as this can damage them and cause them to break.

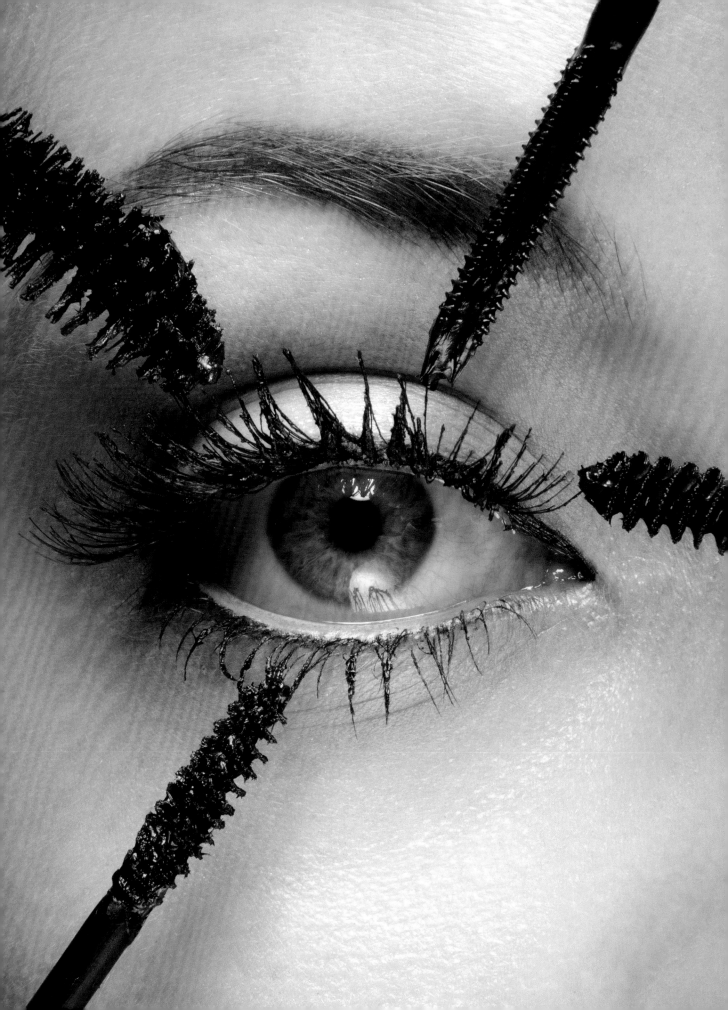

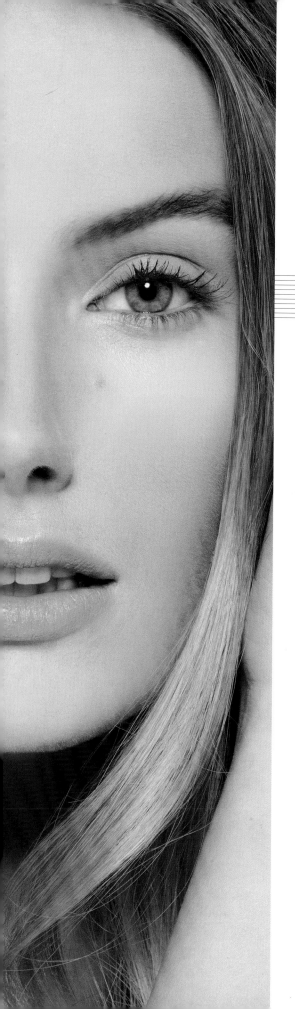

apply mascara like a pro

While it is true that volumizing mascaras, for example, do contain tiny fibers that adhere to the lashes and make them appear thicker (the downside is that they can flake), I find that the end result is largely down to application technique.

Classic daytime lashes

I like to apply mascara to both sides of the top lashes. First, looking down, sweep the wand along the top of the lashes from the lash line to the tips. Open your eye and take the wand underneath the lashes, zigzagging the brush along their length from roots to tips to lift them up. Comb through the tips to separate them. With what's left on the wand, gently zigzag over the bottom lashes to give them some color.

PRO TRICKS

\# Curl your lashes right at the roots. Then use waterproof mascara to set the curl: press the wand into the roots and gently work it from side to side, but don't take it up to the ends. Use your regular mascara on the tips of your lashes to keep them fluttery and light with all the volume at the root.

\# For a soft-looking, smudgeproof finish, use dark brown waterproof mascara on your bottom lashes and top it off with regular mascara in dark brown or black on your top lashes.

LASH EXTENSIONS

Lash extensions are a salon treatment in which individual false lashes are attached to your own lashes to create length and thickness; they will need to be infilled every two to three weeks at the salon. Lash extensions are a great option for those worried about very sparse lashes or sudden lash loss due to medical treatments, but over time it can put a strain on your natural lashes.

Luxe nighttime lashes

For added glamour, layer on more product at the roots: this is the best way to create volume. Hold the wand vertically and use the end to press the product up into the roots of the lashes, working all the way along the lash line. Use a metal comb, which is more precise than a plastic one, to remove any clumps from the tips of the lashes—combing them all the way through will just remove all the product you have applied. Volume at the roots is fine, but you want the ends to be separated and fluttery.

WATERPROOF MASCARA

On the plus side, waterproof mascara is extremely long-wearing, smudge- and tearproof. The downside is that it is difficult to take off and you don't want to scrub the delicate eye area. Soak two cotton pads in oil-based cleanser and hold it over your closed eyes for about 30 seconds to let it dissolve the mascara, then very gently wipe the lashes clean.

Top tip For the most natural, barely-there daytime look, you can either have your lashes professionally tinted—the low-maintenance option—or use a waterproof lash tint. Both of these are great for the beach, gym, swimming, and emotional occasions.

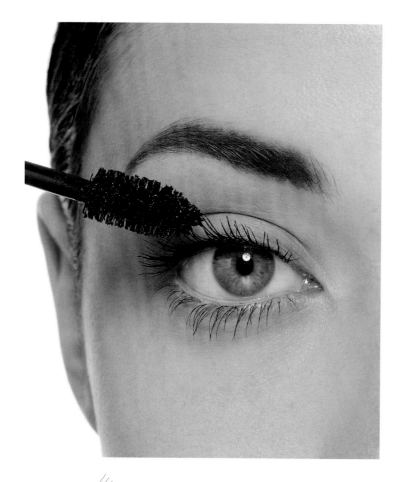

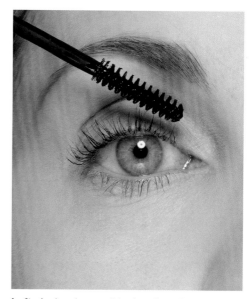

Left A classic conditioning, lengthening, and thickening mascara is flattering for everyone.
Above Tint gives a very natural finish, dries faster, and lasts longer than regular mascara.

I believe you can create any effect with any mascara—it all depends on how much product you put on and your technique

WHAT TO DO IF YOU HAVE...

Very fair lashes Make a lash tint part of your routine to give you a foundation of color. You can then add volume and definition with mascara.

Short lashes Curl the lashes right at the roots, then apply lots of volumizing mascara to the roots and keep the ends fluttery to give the impression of long lashes.

Long or straight lashes Curl the lashes in three steps: at the roots, midway along, and right at the tips. Then add lashings of mascara.

Sparse lashes Use the tightlining technique (see page 52) to create the impression of a fuller, deeper lash line. You can also use eyeliner to fill in any gaps between the lashes and lightly dust them with fine, matte powder to add volume. Then concentrate on building lots of mascara onto the lashes, holding the wand vertically and working it from roots to tips.

The type of brush has a part to play, but results also depend on the formula of the mascara. Formulas that add length and volume contain larger particles that build up and bulk out the lashes.

1   The curved brush fits the shape of the eye, enabling the lashes to be curled, fanned out, and volumized.

2   Small bristles coat even the tiniest hairs, giving volume to the lashes.

3   Plastic bristles allow you to build up the product and separate the lashes, giving length, volume, and definition, with no clumping.

4   The slim brush separates the lashes and applies a light coat of lash tint that can be built up to achieve the desired volume and length.

5   This brush uses V-Groove technology, enabling it to pick up the product and distribute it onto the lashes quickly, for fast volume.

6   The long bristles on this curved brush distribute lots of product quickly, giving volume, lift, and curl.

MAGIC WANDS

Classic bristle-brush wands are good for getting lots of mascara into the roots and building up layers on the lashes. The natural bristles also get between fine, short lashes better.

Plastic silicone wands give precise definition to the lashes, but they do tend to clump up very fine lashes. The formulation doesn't absorb into the wand, so there is more product to coat your lashes, giving an instant result.

Globe or dome-topped wands have bristles that go all the way over the tip, so they are really good for getting into corners.

Small precision brushes are great for applying mascara to corner lashes and fine bottom lashes.

FALSE LASHES

Falsies are a great way to add instant thickness, volume, length, or decoration to your lashes on a temporary basis. You can keep them looking as natural as possible or make a dramatic fashion statement.

From individual lashes that give a very subtle boost to the length and volume of your natural lashes, to colorful falsies adorned with crystals, glitter, or feathers, there are endless false-lash options to enhance your natural flutter.

Curl your natural lashes before applying false ones and work eyeliner into the roots and along the lash line to help hide the join.

Individual lashes

Lash clusters let you create tailor-made lashes to suit your eyes. They come in three or four lengths and you can apply as many or as few as you wish.

How to apply: Put a dab of lash glue on the back of your hand. Pick up the lash cluster with tweezers and dip the roots in the glue. Looking straight into the mirror, drop the root of the cluster onto the roots of your lashes, following the curve of your own lashes. Add them where you want extra volume and length, but keep the longest ones on the outer corners, graduating to the shorter ones near the inner corners.

Corner lashes

Creating definition and drama at the outer corner of the eyes, corner lashes are great accessories for a flick. They are really easy to put on and take off and you can layer them to create a variety of looks.

How to apply: Grasp the tip of the corner lashes with tweezers and apply a small amount of glue along the base. Wait for 20 seconds until the glue is tacky, then place the lashes along the roots of the natural lashes at the outer corner of the eye, making sure the outer corner is slightly lifted.

Full lashes

There is a plethora of full-lash shapes on the market that will enable you to create everything from a soft, wispy look to a dramatic vintage eye.

How to apply: If the false lashes are too wide for your eyes, trim them to fit. Pick the lashes up at the tip with tweezers. Apply a small amount of glue along the base and a little way along the false lashes themselves. Wait for 20 seconds until the glue is tacky, then position the lashes at the center of your lash line. When the glue has adhered, take the inner corner of the lashes with your tweezers and guide it into place. Repeat for the outer corner. Squeeze the lashes between your finger and thumb all the way along.

Fashion lashes

Brands such as Shu Uemura have beautiful limited-edition lashes adorned with feathers, glitter, crystals—you name it. These are great fun for a special party or fancy dress.

How to apply: Use the same method as for full lashes (see above).

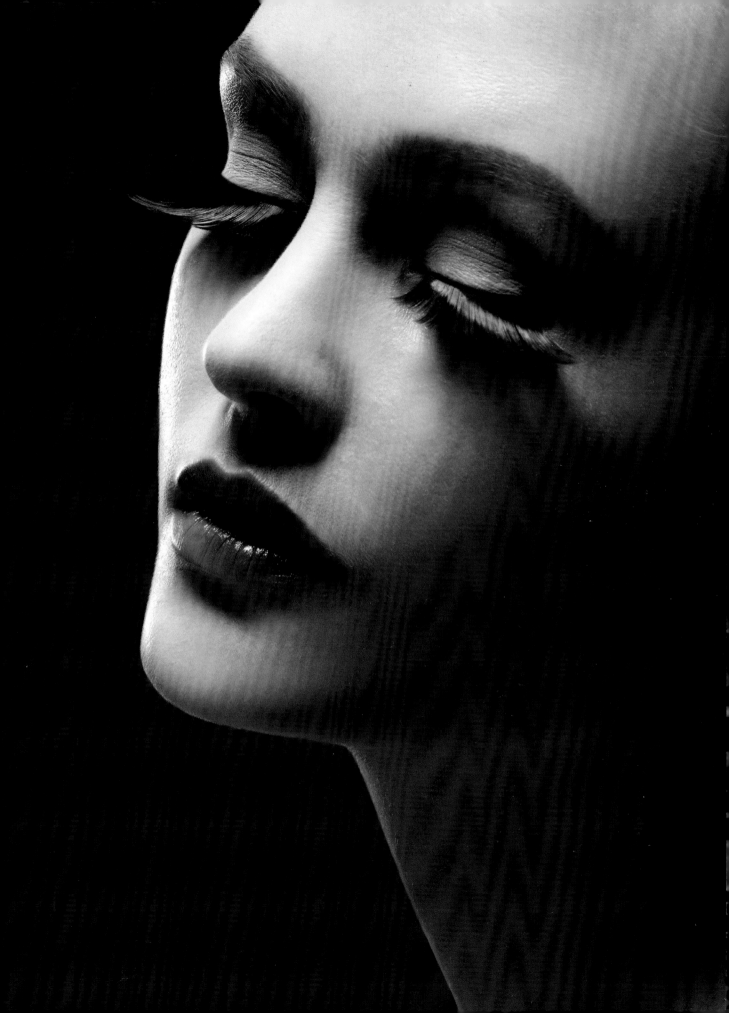

HOW TO REMOVE FALSE LASHES

Soak a cotton pad with eye-make-up remover. Close your eye and hold the pad over it, pressing gently for a few seconds to soften the glue. Starting at the outer corner, gently peel the false lashes away. Clean off the glue—stubborn glue can be removed with sweet almond oil—and put the lashes back in their box. If you look after your false lashes, you can use them numerous times.

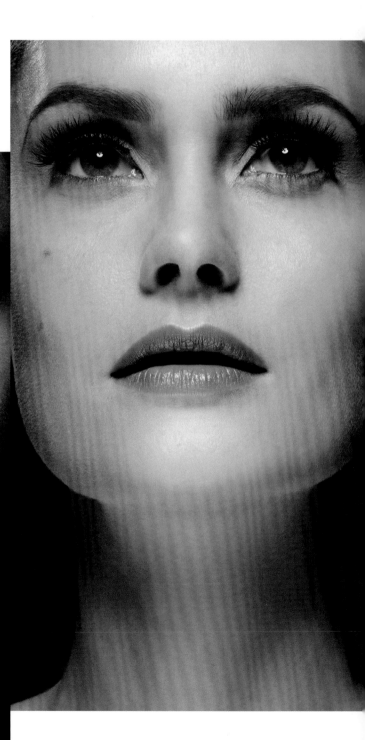

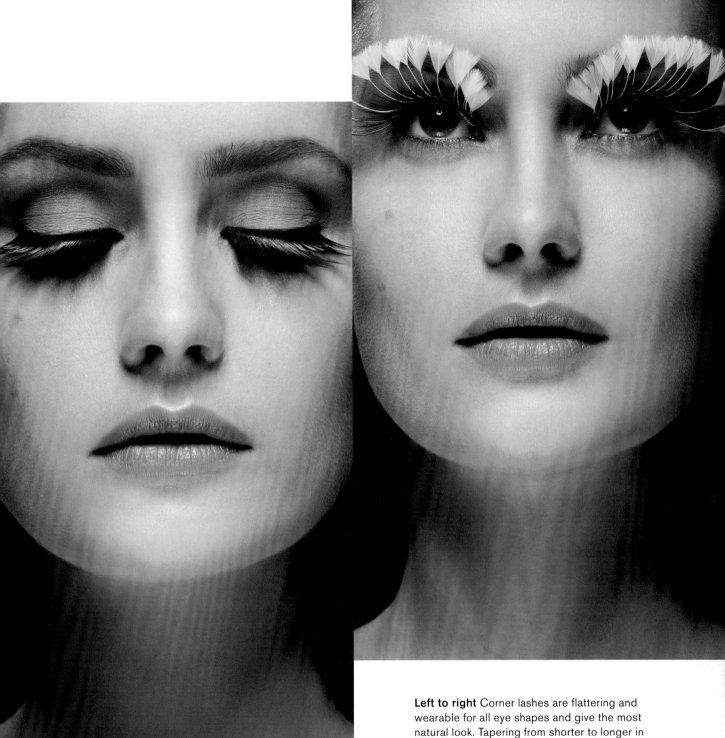

Left to right Corner lashes are flattering and wearable for all eye shapes and give the most natural look. Tapering from shorter to longer in the outer corners, they elongate the eyes and add length and thickness to the lashes. Full lashes are less subtle and can be tricky to wear in the daytime, but the drama they create is fantastic for a big event. Choose false lashes on cotton thread rather than nylon, as cotton sits flatter along the lash line. The focus should be on the outer part of the eyes, so don't position them too close to the inner corners of the eyes. Fashion lashes, such as these fabulous feathered examples, are pure fun. Elaborately decorative, extreme lashes make a statement and are great for parties and fancy dress.

BROWS

Brows are the finishing touch and when you do them everything comes together. Well-groomed brows frame your face and their power to polish your look should never be underestimated.

Correctly shaped brows can take years off you, as they lift the entire face and make your eyes look bigger. If you have never had your brows shaped professionally, go to a brow specialist or a brow bar and have them threaded or waxed—you will be amazed by the difference it makes. Once you have the most flattering brow shape for your face, you just need to maintain it.

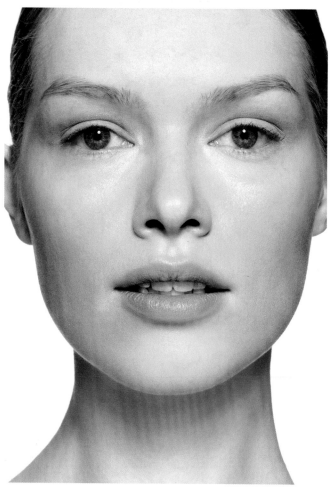

the perfect brow shape

The highest part of the arch (2) should be about two-thirds of the way along the eye from the inner corner (1). The brow should always start just before the eyes and not after, but make sure it doesn't start too low or close to your nose, as that will look heavy and give the impression of a frown.

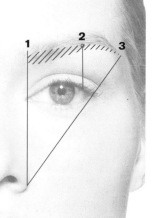

The aim is that the inner part of the brow should slope gently upward to the highest point of the arch and then taper down toward the outer corner (3), which should be the lowest point of the eyebrow.

GOLDEN RULE

Never overpluck, as it makes the area between the socket and the browbone look too heavy and gives you an expression of permanent surprise. Overplucking is also aging and can create unevenness and holes where the hairs never grow back, which make brows look unkempt. Thick brows are more youthful, so embrace a bushy brow, but keep it tidy. As we age, hair thins and brows get sparse, so think ahead and don't overpluck.

Don't interfere with your brows too much. Once you have the shape you like, simply maintain it by plucking out any stray hairs to keep your brows nice and neat.

This is the same girl, with the same make-up and lighting —the only difference is the brow. The groomed and colored brow makes her look instantly more tailored and sophisticated with wider eyes. This transformation was achieved using my Brow Kit. First, the brows were brushed into a good shape. Then, using an angled brush and a brow powder one shade lighter than her natural brows to create a shadow effect, the brows were filled in and the arch emphasized two-thirds of the way across, before tapering the brow down to a point and blending the powder well so there are no hard lines.

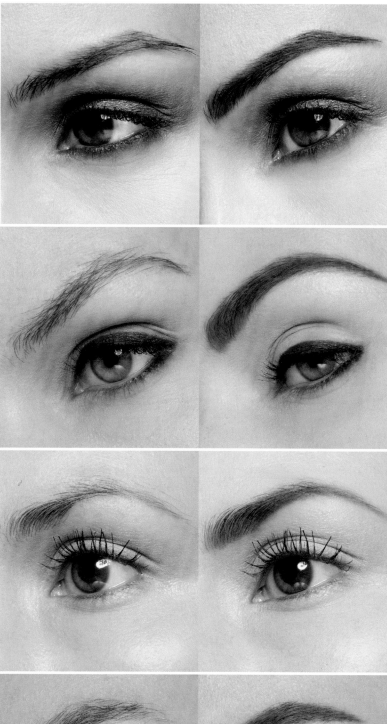

STRAIGHT BROW
The brow is naturally quite straight, so make-up was used to thicken and lift it, giving it more of an arch. The brow was reshaped with a pencil and then brow powder was blended on top for a natural, feathery look. The end of the brow near the nose and underneath this area was darkened and thickened, then two-thirds of the way along, the make-up was taken just above the brow to create an arch.

ARCHED BROW
This brow started off with a nice shape, but it was gappy and uneven, so the aim was to fill it in to give a smoother shape and extend the tail to elongate the eye. The brow was simply colored in along its natural shape, following the arch, and the tail was extended slightly. Highlighter was applied just underneath the arch to lift it and create a sharper, more tailored finish.

TADPOLE BROW
This is a classic brow shape that results from overplucking. The only hairs left are the ones near the bridge of the nose and they taper off to almost nothing. The heavy end over the nose gives the impression of a frown and is something to avoid, especially if you have close-set eyes. The aim was to thicken up the tail of the brow to balance it, by deepening the color and coming just below the natural brow line. As always, the highest part of the brow was created two-thirds of the way along.

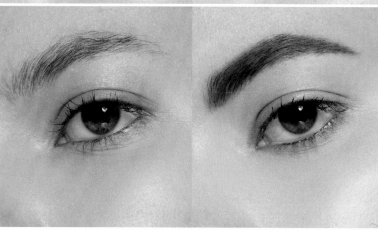

SPARSE BROW
This short, sparse brow is almost the opposite of the tadpole, as it had lost all of its depth at the bridge of the nose, was thicker in the middle, and then tapered out again. Color was applied at the bridge of the nose and blended out into the thicker part of the brow, so as not to make that part any heavier. The color was then blended out to the outer corner for a tapered effect.

TOP TIPS

Pluck from the root, one hair and line at a time, working from under the brows.

Grasp the hair firmly with the tweezers and pull in the direction of growth.

When applying brow make-up, blend the color evenly and keep the edges soft.

If you are using a pencil, brush the brows up with a mascara wand or brow brush for a natural finish.

If you dye your hair, make sure the color of your brows is not too much of a contrast.

brow make-up
Whether you use brow powder, pencil, or a mascara-like brow shaper, don't go any darker than your natural brow color. You may find that one shade lighter works best, because once the product goes on the hair it will automatically look darker.

Brow powders, which should be applied with a thin, angled brush to give control and precision, are my make-up of choice for natural groomed brows. Powder enables you to improve the shape of the brows by brushing them into place while darkening and coating the hairs, and you can blend it easily to create a natural feathery finish that looks like real hair. It is the best product to use to fill in any gaps, because it blends so naturally.

Brow pencils work well on thinner brows, where you want a harder defining line. The Brow Perfector in my range comes in brown and blonde shades, each with a main color crayon and a brow-lift highlighter. The crayon should be used to shape and shade the brows, while the highlighter should be applied right under the roots of the bottom line of hairs to frame the colored area and create "lift."

Wax sealers hold onto the hairs and keep them in place. I find these work best on shorter, thinner brows.

INSIDER SECRETS

Brow expert Shavata shares her top 10 tips for perfect brows:

1 You need a good pair of tweezers and an eyebrow brush—you are as good as your tools.

2 Don't try to wax or thread your own brows—only ever use tweezers on yourself.

3 Use a large mirror to pluck your eyebrows so that you can see both at the same time. Have a magnifying mirror on hand for a close-up view.

4 If you find it easier, draw your desired brow shape with a brow pencil and then pluck away the hairs around this shape.

5 It is much easier to get your brows even if you work on both eyebrows simultaneously, taking a few hairs from one and then the other. If you get one perfect and then try to copy it, you may struggle to get them both the same.

6 Eyebrows are sisters not twins—your eyebrows will be naturally different and it is impossible to get them exactly the same.

7 If you make a mistake while plucking, don't try to correct it—you will only make the problem worse. Instead, use a brow pencil to fill in the gap until the hair grows back.

8 Never pluck a week before or during your period, as the skin is more sensitive and it will be more painful.

9 Don't fight nature: work with what you have. Everybody has different eyebrows, so style your brows to suit your lifestyle, personality, look, age, and the type of make-up you wear. This will make maintenance easier, too—for example, if you have thick, bushy brows, plucking them thin will leave you with a lot of regrowth to deal with.

10 Nobody should ever see make-up on your brows—they should look completely natural.

THE
EYE

SMOKY

This is one of the most popular make-up applications and is never out of fashion. Whether you make it sexy, sultry, classic, or contemporary, the smoky eye is incredibly flattering for all eye shapes.

The smoky eye is a true classic and one of my favorite evening looks.

Smoky eyes are always thought of as black, but the term really refers to the effect—that lovely graduation of color intensity. This is due to the application technique, which creates the signature smoky softness around the eyes where the intense color has been blended out and tapers off to nothing.

I wanted to show how versatile this effect can be. While black is the classic and most popular color, especially for nighttime, smoky eyes look fantastic in many other hues, too—from purple and green to gray and brown, which works well in the day. Traditionally, this look was always done using powder eyeshadows, but now you can use creams, mousses, crayons, or even some eyeliners, or a combination of formulas that can be blended with your finger, sponge applicators, or brushes. This makes it really easy to achieve matte, pearl, or wet smoky looks.

EVERYDAY BROWN SMOKY EYES

A daytime smoky eye shouldn't be too strong, so no eyeliner was used and the application of the soft pearl eyeshadows in graduating shades of brown, from bitter chocolate to creamy mocha, was kept light and subtle.

CLASSIC BLACK SMOKY EYES

This is the quintessential smoky eye—the perfect nighttime look that goes with everything and works for any occasion, from drinks or dinners to parties and formal occasions. The color is strongest by the roots of the lashes and tapers out to just under the browbone, like a soft, smoky cloud. A defined brow is essential to balance the look and frame the eyes.

ROCK CHICK SMOKY EYES

This is where all of your make-up techniques are thrown out of the window. I love a cream base because it gives a wet, watery, glossy finish that catches the light and seems fluid. This isn't a difficult look to do, but it is messy and high-maintenance.

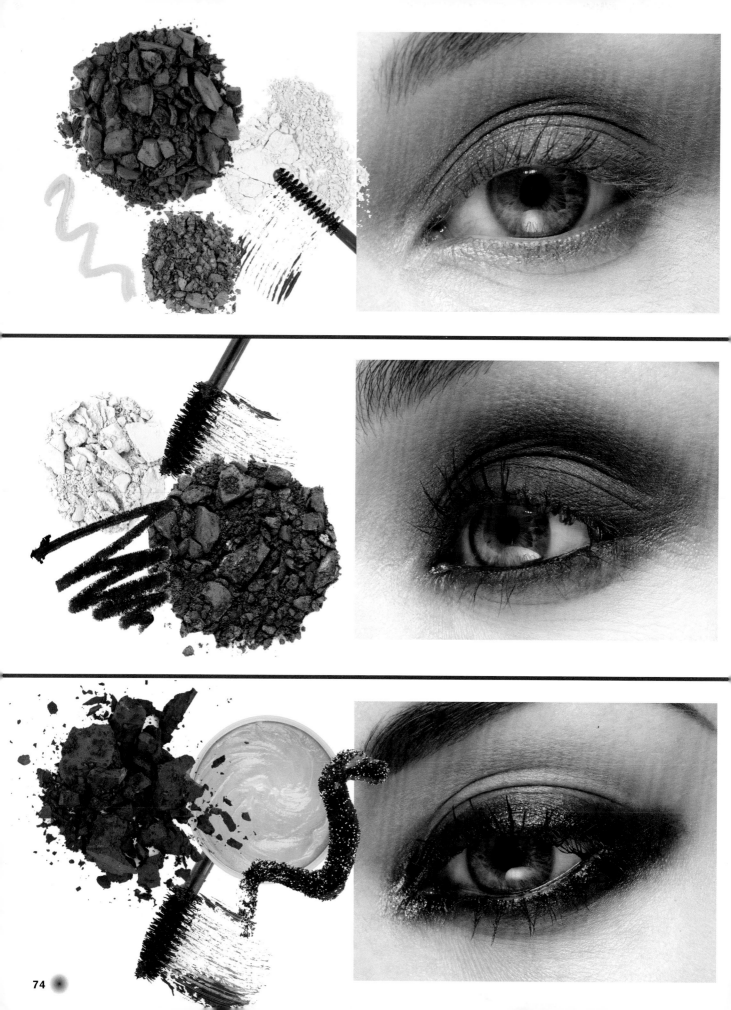

EVERYDAY BROWN SMOKY EYES

1 Use an eye primer on the mobile lid. This holds the pigment, giving instant color, and provides a good, creamy base for blending the eyeshadows to a soft finish.

2 With a small, flat brush, apply dark brown eyeshadow along the upper and lower lash lines.

3 Blend soft pearl mocha eyeshadow on top and then over the mobile lid. Because of the primer, you should get an even finish very quickly. With a socket brush, blend the color above the crease so that when the eye is open you can see the color fading in intensity up toward the browbone.

4 For a really soft finish, brush a little bone-colored or translucent powder along the browbone to give the color something to blend into. Make sure there are no hard lines above the crease, or it will look like panda eyes.

5 Dust a little loose powder under the lower lash line to balance it out and keep it soft.

6 Apply one light coat of lengthening black mascara and define your brows.

CLASSIC BLACK SMOKY EYES

1 Prep and prime the eyes to neutralize any redness and provide a creamy base for the eyeshadow to adhere to. Brush a little bone-colored or translucent powder under the brow and over the upper part of the lid above the crease line and just underneath the lower lash line for easy blending.

2 Apply pitch-black pencil eyeliner over the inner rims and upper lash line, working between the roots of the lashes. Take the pencil from the upper lash line onto the lid itself and blend it with your finger. This will create a dark base for the eyeshadow and intensify its pigment.

3 Apply dark gray eyeshadow over the whole lid and up to the crease line, blending it to just under the brow using small circular motions to give a really soft smoky finish.

4 Blend the color underneath the lower lash line, making sure you get that really soft finish.

5 Go over the inner rims, upper lash line, and between the roots of the lashes again with the eyeliner.

6 Curl the lashes, apply black mascara, and darken the brow to frame the eyes.

ROCK CHICK SMOKY EYES

1 Use a synthetic brush or your finger to blend black cream all around the rim of the eyes, emphasizing the inner and outer corners to create impact. You don't need to come up above the crease line at all here—just darken the mobile lid and push the color out horizontally from the outer corner of the eye.

2 Dab a little black powder on the outer corners of the eyes to set the cream and prevent it from sliding. Note: If you can't find black cream, use a petroleum-based lip balm such as Vaseline, and press black powder pigment into it and blend well.

3 Define and darken the brows and highlight the browbones with bone-colored powder.

4 Apply lashings of mascara. Make sure the wand is packed full of product—you want lumps and clumps so the lashes look spidery and full.

5 Go over the inner rims of the eyes with black eyeliner.

6 Finish by applying black glitter gel liner along the upper lash line to catch the light.

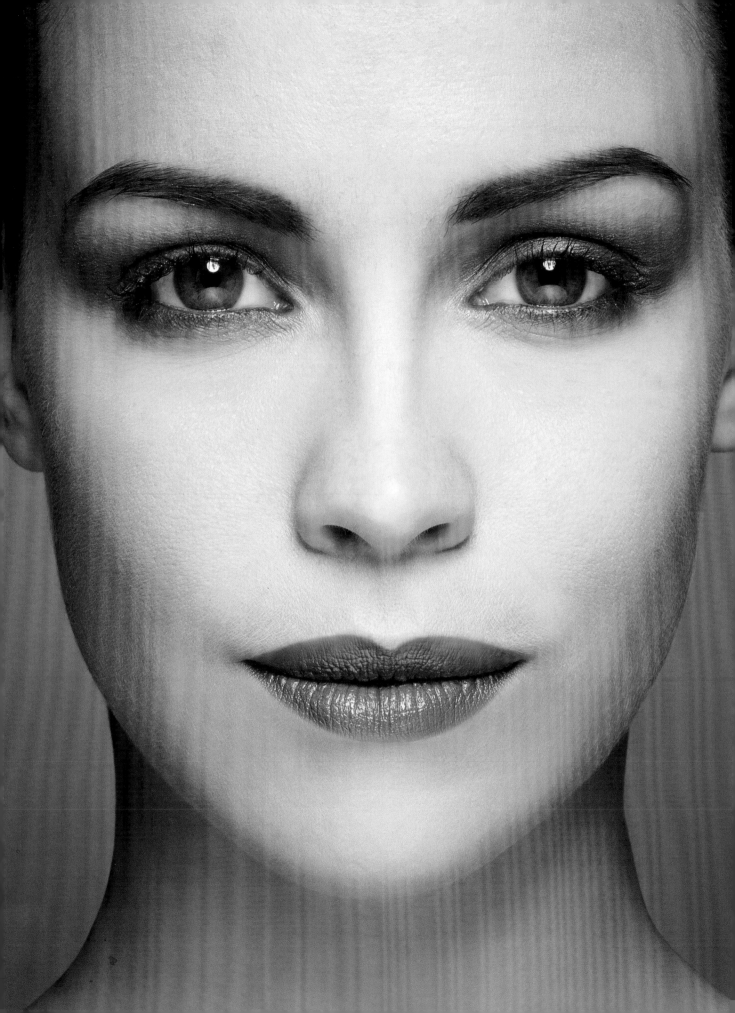

COLOR WARDROBES

Here are some of the most popular color palettes for eyes and how to wear them. Don't be afraid of color—it doesn't have to be bold, you can just rock a dash of colored liner or a subtle colorwash. These are versatile hues, with shades to suit every skin tone.

The more vibrant yellow golds work best as a highlighter.
Metallic and glitter golds are great for parties.
If you have green eyes, try gold with purple or red tones.
If you have blue eyes, orange-based gold will make them pop.

gold

There are many shades of gold, with yellow, green, brown, or orange undertones, ranging from a soft pearl finish to a metallic or glitter pigment. It is a matter of finding the one that suits you best.

Get the look

This is a blending exercise of gold and brown, a combination that is incredibly flattering and wearable. After prepping the eye to neutralize any redness, apply a dull yellow-toned gold over the central part of the lid, without taking it all the way to the corners. Then blend a rich warm brown from the outer corner of the eye along the socket in an arc and down to the inner corner. This accentuates the socket and frames the gold, making it come forward. Work brown pencil eyeliner into the roots

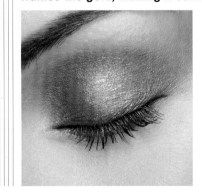

of the lashes to define the eyes. Use a smudger to ensure there are no hard lines and then pat a little brown eyeshadow on top to seal it and soften the edges. Curl the lashes and apply mascara, then groom the brows to frame the eyes.

A bold berry mouth complements the gold eyes, with a slight clash that helps it to pop. Pat the lipstick onto your lips with your forefinger to give a semi-stain finish. Warm up the cheeks with pale apricot blush.

WHICH SHADE?

All shades of gold suit warm-toned olive skin.

The deeper your skin tone, the richer you can go— all the way to the orange-based golds.

Yellow- and green-based golds are best for pale skin.

Warm brown golds suit all but very porcelain skin.

The most wearable shades are the soft pearl richer, greener "old" golds.

brown

The safest and most wearable of all eyeshadows, brown is the color that sells the best because it gives the most natural look and is also perfect for shading and contouring. Brown has no contrast, so it goes with everything and works with all skin tones.

Get the look

Apply a rich, muddy brown eyeshadow to the lids, taking it up to the socket line, then blend it up and out to give a soft hue of color like an aura—mimic the eyebrow shape, blending the color up toward the arch of the brow. This shading makes the eyes look bigger. Use a small brush to dab eyeshadow onto the lower lash line at the outer corners and blend it to about one-third of the way along. Use a flesh-colored eyeliner on the inner rims. Blend a touch of warm camel eyeshadow into the inner corners of the eyes and along the browbone. Groom the brows, curl the lashes, and apply lots of mascara.
The eyes were complemented with a warm-toned dirty pink blush on the cheeks and a natural nude balm on the lips.

Everyone loves black eyeliner, but I think brown eyeliner is more flattering and wearable, especially as we age. Keep the lid pale with bone-colored eyeshadow and a little shading in the socket line to open up the eye. Apply brown pencil eyeliner along the upper lash line, following its shape. Concentrate on the upper lid but apply a little to the lower lash line, depending on your eye shape.

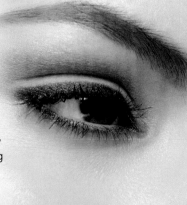

Gold- and copper-toned browns work well on warm skin tones.

Raw, earthy, dirty browns that contain more green than orange are the most flattering and can be used all over the face for shading and contouring.

Yellow- or orange-based browns make blue eyes pop; red- or plum-based browns make green eyes pop.

Soft pink-based browns work well on porcelain and cool fair skin.

natural

Stealth make-up is all about looking like you, but better, using natural colors that blend with the skin—soft camels, taupes, light browns, and pinks. It is the perfect day look, but it is harder to do than it looks, because it is all about subtle contouring and blending.

Get the look

Work a soft neutral taupe, a couple of shades deeper than the skin tone, over the lid. Blend a slightly deeper color into the socket. Add a touch of soft pearl highlighter under the brows and blend it all really well so there are no hard lines and the washes of color merge together. Blend a little of the taupe eyeshadow right under the lower lash lines to give the eyes depth. Curl the lashes and apply a dark brown lash tint. Neaten the brows and fill in any gaps.

A cream blush in a powdery pink blended over the apple of the cheeks keeps the skin looking very real. Finish with a soft pink lipstick.

Barely-there make-up appears effortless, but it takes time to do well and requires skillful blending for a perfect natural look

WHICH SHADE?

Choose shades that complement your skin tone. If you have warm skin, go for yellow- and orange-based beige, taupe, and light browns; if you have cool skin, choose nudes with pink undertones.

Use very soft shades with a light pearl finish to make the skin look radiant—nothing too matte or too much of a highlighter.

plum

plum Tones include everything from violet, lilac, amethyst, and lavender to deep purples and eggplant. Plum can be worn as a bold or accent color, blended with gray or brown, or as an eyeliner for a more subtle look.

Get the look

Prime the face and eye area well, as the red tone will accentuate any redness, while the purple will emphasize undereye circles. Use a plum pencil eyeliner along the top and bottom lash lines and blend away any hard edges. Apply the lilac eyeshadow over the lid and blend it upward and outward. Don't overcomplicate the make-up, so the color really sings. Groom the brows to frame the face, curl the lashes, and apply lots of black mascara.

A touch of peach blush and nude lips ensure that nothing detracts from the statement eyes.

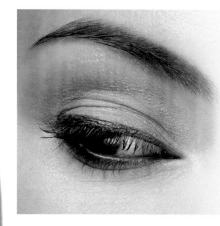

Apply a wash of neutral eyeshadow over the lid, with a touch of shading in the socket to deepen it. Frame the eye along the top lash line with purple eyeliner and then, using a small brush, dab powder eyeshadow on top to deepen the color. Curl the lashes and apply black mascara.

WHICH SHADE?

\# Cooler lavender tones look good on paler skin.

\# Deep, rich plums look better on warm skin tones.

\# Mix purple with black for a bold evening look, and plum with brown for the daytime—combining any color with black or brown makes it more wearable. Try a mid-plum over the center of the lid with an arc of soft brown blended into the socket.

green

Depending on the shade and finish, green can be worn as a statement or toned down for everyday. Deeper, brown-based greens in a matte to soft pearl finish are the most wearable shades, while bright greens and metallic finishes are for the bold and brave.

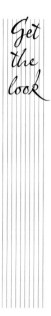

Get the look

Apply black eyeliner along the lash lines, focusing on the outer corners. Brush deep olive eyeshadow over the lid and blend it upward and outward, but don't take it beyond the socket crease. Dab black eyeshadow over the eyeliner on the top and bottom lash lines and blend it for a soft, shadowy finish. Blend a little black eyeshadow into the socket crease, focusing on the outer corner to frame the green with soft gray. Add a touch of highlighter under the browbones. Groom the brows, curl the lashes, and apply black mascara. Warm the cheeks with neutral taupe blush and keep the lips nude, so that it is all about the eyes and nothing clashes with the green.

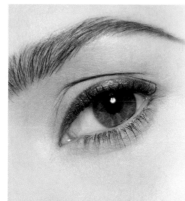

For the most wearable look, you need nothing more than primer on the eye and green pencil eyeliner along the upper lash line. Curl your lashes and add black mascara.

WHICH SHADE?

\#   Earthy olive is a flattering shade for most skin tones.

\#   Combining green with black or brown tones it down and makes it instantly more wearable.

\#   Metallic finishes, bright hues, and liquid liners work well for a fun party look if you are young.

silver

True blue-toned silver is a color to use on cool skin—it looks beautiful on porcelain and fair skin but will clash with warmer tones. Here, silver cream gives a wash of color all over the eyes.

Get the look

Apply the cream over the mobile lid, ensuring you get a smooth, even finish, and don't take it above the socket. Using a brush, pat silver eyeshadow into the cream to set it, and blend it out. Apply black eyeliner along the upper lash line, following the shape of the eye. Work it between the lashes to make them look thicker. Darken the brow with powder—you need the definition of the brow and eyeliner to help frame the eyes. Curl the lashes and apply mascara. Keep the face pretty and fresh, with a little pale pink blush and soft pink lipstick.

Black eyeliner has to be a sharp, neat line, whereas silver eyeliner just highlights the eye. Simply dab it along the upper lash line to create a soft, smudgy line. This is a pretty look for cool-toned girls, but you can do the same with gold eyeliner if your skin is warm. Beware, though, if you have any lines or wrinkles on your lid, this will highlight them.

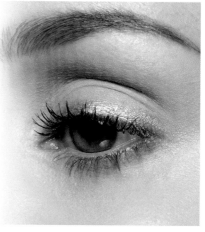

WHICH SHADE?

\# Cool blue-toned slates and silvery grays suit those with cool skin.

\# Warm taupe-grays and soft charcoal flatter warm skin.

\# Grays are equally glamorous and sultry in shimmery metallics and soft matte finishes.

gray and black

This is a favorite combination for classic smoky eyes and, when done well, nothing can beat it. Thorough blending is essential to get that lovely soft shading around the socket.

Get the look

Blend black pencil eyeliner into the roots of the lashes and along the lash lines and inner rims. Start at the inner corner of the top lash line and work to the outer corner, making a subtle flick. Then work back along the lower lash line. Dot the pencil between the lashes and then blend it with a smudger. Apply slate-gray eyeshadow over the eyeliner and lid. Work the color into the socket, blending it up and out, following the eye shape to create an elongated tail that accentuates the outer corners. Apply highlighter above the socket and blend it into the gray. Then go over the rim of the eye again with eyeliner to make it the darkest area. Curl the lashes and apply lots of black mascara—the darker and gloopier, the better. Add corner lashes or individual false lashes for extra fullness and length.
Use a soft brownish blush a couple of shades deeper than the skin—more like a contour color. Keep the lips a warm nude with a touch of gloss—nothing that detracts from the eyes.

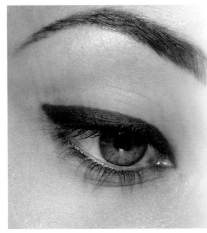

A natural eye can be given instant definition with black eyeliner. Draw a thick line along the upper lash line and flick it slightly up and out at the outer corners to elongate the eyes. Make sure you get right into the roots of the lashes and blend it well for an even finish.

★ **Top tip** Shape the brow and darken it—you need a strong brow to frame a strong eye.

The 10 most-asked questions about eyes

1

How can I make my eyes look bigger?

The best way to do this is to deepen and elongate the socket line. What makes eyes look smaller is when loose skin above the eye covers the eyelid, which makes the upper part of the eye very heavy. To make your eyes look bigger, you need to highlight the eyelid, minimize the fleshy part of the upper lid, and add shading to create a socket and elongate the eye. Apply a pale, soft pearl eyeshadow to the mobile lid to bring it forward. Then use a toning darker color on the area above, blending it up and out to make the fleshy part of the upper lid recede and give the illusion of a socket. Curl the lashes to open up the eyes more, and darken the lashes and their roots to make them look fuller.

2

How can I prevent my eyeshadow from creasing?

The best way to ensure that eyeshadow doesn't crease and lasts longer is to use an eye primer underneath it. Stay away from cream eyeshadow, as this creases more easily than powder shadows. You can also get high-pigment liquid colorwashes for your eyes, which dry on your eyelid and hold the pigment like a paint or a stain.

4

What are the best colors for my eyes?

Brown eyes look good in most shades of eyeshadow, as brown doesn't have a contrast color.

Blue eyes are enhanced by cool blues, grays, slates, and ashy taupes. The contrast to blue is orange, so to pop blue eyes wear ocher or orange-toned eyeshadows, camel tones, and rich browns.

Green eyes look great in camel tones, taupes, browns, and moss colors. The contrast to green is red, so to pop green eyes wear purple, red, or pink tones.

Hazel eyes will be enhanced by camels, taupes, and browns. The contrast to orange is blue, so to pop the orange flecks in hazel eyes, wear shades of blue, navy, and blue-toned slates. To pop the green flecks, see above.

3

How can I stop my mascara from smudging?

Experiment with different formulations to find one that is right for your eyes. Try waterproof, long-wear or smudgeproof mascara or a lash tint. Don't be wary of waterproof mascara, as modern formulations are much less drying and easier to take off than they used to be. If you rub your eyes a lot, it is your best option. Or try using waterproof mascara on the bottom lashes and a regular volumizing and thickening mascara on the top lashes.

5

My eye area is crepy—what can I do?

Algae is a natural skin tightener, so look for it in your eye cream or serum. If you have any crepiness around your eyes, stay away from anything metallic or any product that has a highlighting effect, and stick with matte to pearl finishes. Prep the eye area well before making up your eyes (see page 44), then make the crepy undereye area disappear by using a warm apricot-toned ultrafine powder to push it back.

6

What is the best way to correct mistakes?

Use a Q-tip dipped in make-up remover to wipe away the mistake. You can also buy special eye-make-up correctors, which come impregnated with cleanser and ready to use. Then apply a dab of skin-brightening apricot-toned color corrector or foundation and use the other end of the Q-tip to blend it seamlessly.

7

What can I do if my eyes look tired?

Redness around the eyes is aging and makes you look tired, so use a concealer or a product like my I-Perfector, and line the inner rims of the eyes with a flesh-colored eyeliner. This takes away redness and instantly opens up the eyes, making them appear bigger, brighter, and more wide awake.

8

What brushes do I need for my eye make-up?

Use soft natural-bristle brushes for powder products, as they blend better; use stiffer synthetic brushes for cream products, as they give more control and precision and won't absorb the product like natural brushes do.

A small, square-tipped, short-bristled dense brush is useful for lining the eyes and defining the brows.

Use a medium-sized natural-bristle brush for applying powder eyeshadow and a synthetic one for applying cream shadow.

A natural-bristle smudging brush, cut to fit the shape of the socket, is great for blending and diffusing powder eyeshadow.

A pointed eyeshadow brush is useful for adding detail and for shading under the eye.

9

How should I clean my brushes?

Clean your brushes regularly, especially the ones you use for your eyes, as eyes are far more sensitive and prone to infections and allergies than other areas of the face. Wash them with brush cleanser or a mild shampoo and warm water, working thoroughly between the fibers with your fingers. Rinse them well and squeeze them in a towel, then leave them to air-dry over the side of the bathtub or sink so air can circulate around the bristles.

10

Are there any other eye essentials I should have?

A good-quality pencil sharpener for both fat eye crayons and thin eyeliner pencils.

Lash curlers—I couldn't live without mine. Always curl your lashes before applying mascara.

Metal lash comb—use it to separate the tips of your lashes after applying mascara.

Brow brush and tweezers with slanted tips for keeping eyebrows neat and tidy.

luscious lips

Mouths and lips are sensual and expressive, revealing our mood and showing that we're happy, cross, determined, flirtatious... They are also, of course, how we communicate—and often the parts of our face that people focus on when we're talking to them—and they're how we kiss.

A fully made-up mouth can be the finishing touch to your look and some women feel naked without their signature lipstick. Others prefer to keep lipstick for evenings out and go bare for much of the time, with no more than a slick of moisturizing balm, a natural gloss, or a subtle stain. The choice is yours. It depends on your mood and your personal style. There are so many formulations and finishes in a rainbow of colors—from tinted balms through to stains, glosses, and long-lasting lipsticks—that there is something to suit every woman.

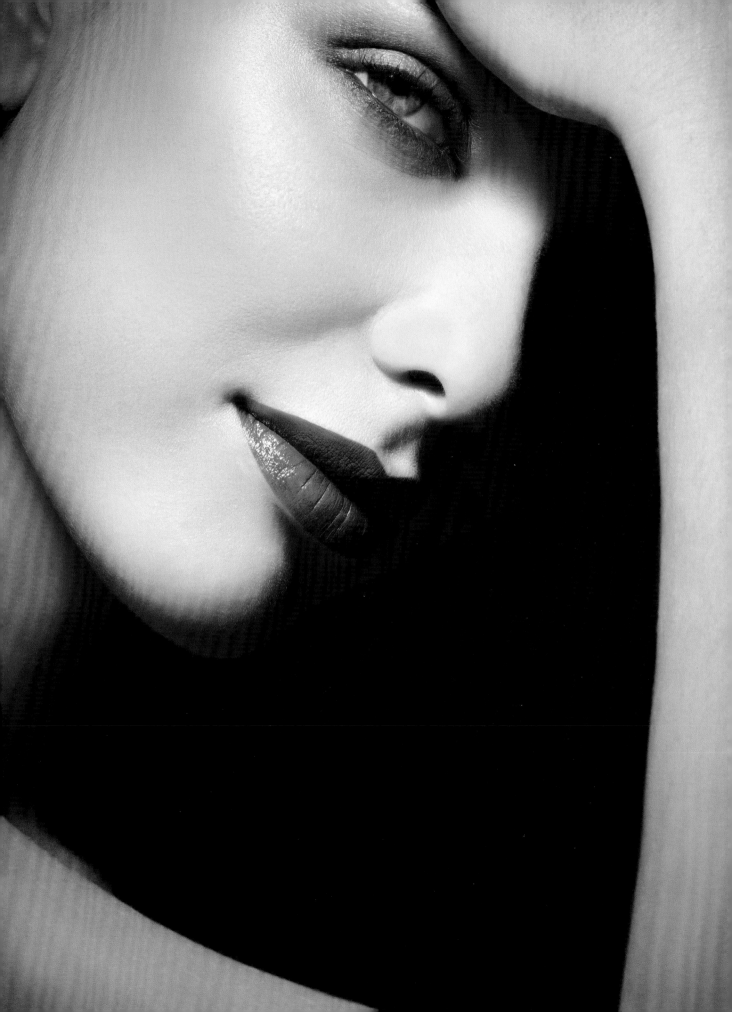

NOURISH AND PROTECT

Whether you can't live without your screen-siren lipstick, prefer a glossy pink pout, or would rather go au naturel with a tinted balm, keeping your lips soft, conditioned, and kissable at all times is paramount.

lip science

The texture of the skin on the lips is completely different from the skin on the rest of the body. It's thinner, made up of only three to five cellular layers whereas typical facial skin comprises up to 16 layers, and it's more sensitive. Lip skin, especially for those with fairer skin tones, contains fewer melanocytes—the cells that create the melanin pigment that gives the skin color—and because of this, blood vessels can be seen through the skin, giving the lips their natural pink hue. The deeper your skin tone, the more melanin in your lip skin, so the less pink your lips will appear. Lip skin has no hair, sweat glands, or sebaceous glands, so it doesn't have the self-protection layer that keeps other skin smooth, which is why we get dry lips.

My mantra

Like an artist, always prep your canvas before you add color.

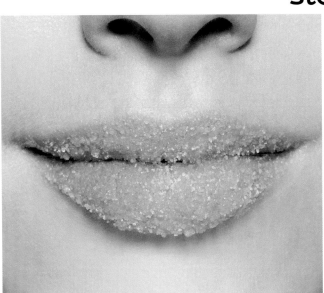

step 1 exfoliate your way to gorgeous lips

Exfoliating is important, especially if you have flaky, chapped lips, which most of us do from time to time because of exposure to the elements—mainly the wind and sun. Removing dry, dead skin regularly is key, not only for revealing a soft, smooth, plump mouth, but also for providing a much better base for adding color—lipstick on chapped lips looks dreadful.

HOW TO EXFOLIATE YOUR LIPS

There are several ways to exfoliate your lips and whichever you choose, be careful not to take away too many layers, or you may end up with a scab.

\# This is my favorite method: apply a little petroleum jelly to your lips with your finger, and then rub them very gently in little circles with a washcloth or a Q-tip.

\# Use a soft toothbrush, working it gently in a circular motion over your lips.

\# Use a special lip exfoliator or sugar scrub. Gently grind it over the skin and then wipe it off with a warm washcloth. You can easily make your own sugar scrub by mixing a little sugar with some olive oil or honey—the drawback is that it tastes very sweet.

step 2 moisturize your way to a plump pout

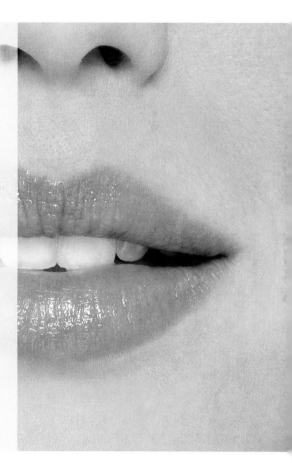

As always, first of all make sure you keep your lips hydrated from the inside by drinking lots of water and then keep them well moisturized with a nourishing balm. I'm a fan of wax-based balms, which really seal in the moisture. Petroleum-based products sit on the surface and, although they may feel good initially, can be drying in the long run. My favorite balms are Burt's Bees Beeswax Lip Balm and Korres Lip Butter.

Top tips ✳ Some lipsticks can be drying because of the concentration of color pigments they contain, especially the long-lasting formulas. If you find this is the case, apply balm under your lipstick to seal in hydration. ✳ Wear SPF at all times, because sun spots around the mouth can ruin its shape. ✳ Try using different lipsticks and glosses so your lips don't get used to one brand.

INGREDIENTS TO LOOK FOR

Beeswax, rice wax, shea butter, plant oils, jojoba oil, nut oils, olive oil, and Vitamin E are all good natural nourishers for lips.

LIP SHAPES

A bit of clever make-up magic can work wonders, creating the illusion of youthfully plump-looking luscious lips, which is what most women long for.

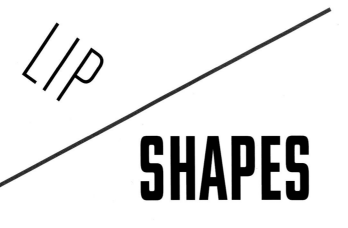

full mouth

A plump pout is nothing but gorgeous and what everyone desires, so if you are lucky enough to have naturally full, cushiony lips, show them off and be proud of them.

Lipstick with a creamy satin texture will make your mouth look really hydrated and moisturized. As a rule, pale colors and glossy finishes will make lips appear even more pouty. Conversely, dark shades and matte textures can be hard to wear, as they tend to make mouths look smaller—but you don't need to worry about that, so have fun and experiment with dramatic colors that catch your eye.

The only word of caution I would offer is to stay away from metallic finishes, as you don't want your mouth to dominate your face or your naturally full lips to look fake.

uneven lips

If, like many women, your bottom lip is fuller than your top lip, it can make you look a little sulky, but some clever trickery with a lip liner is all you need to balance them out. The aim is to plump up the top lip and make the bottom lip look less pouty.

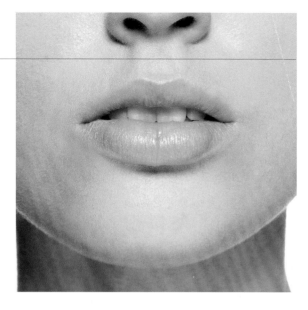

Choose a lip liner that matches your lip tone or the lipstick you are going to use and apply it around the bow only, drawing very slightly above the lip line. Feather it out, so there are no hard lines, but don't take the liner down all the way to the outer corners—you just want to balance the center of the lips, top and bottom, otherwise they will look fake. Then use a little concealer or my Lip Perfector on the bottom part of the bottom lip to tone down the natural color: this will make the bottom lip seem less full.

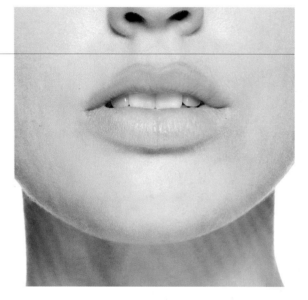

Line the center of the bottom lip a fraction above the natural lip line, feathering it outward, as before, so there are no hard lines. Then pencil in the lower lip so the finish is subtle and not too shiny. Apply matching lipstick to the top lip and a tiny bit to the bottom lip for an even finish. Dab a little gloss onto the center of the upper lip to catch and bounce the light.

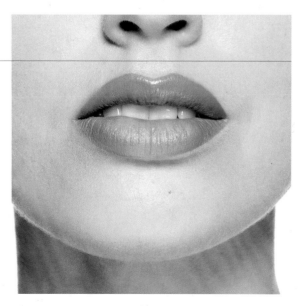

small mouth

If you have a small mouth, it can look too narrow for your face, so the aim is to balance things out by extending the outer corners of the lips to elongate the mouth and make it appear wider on the face.

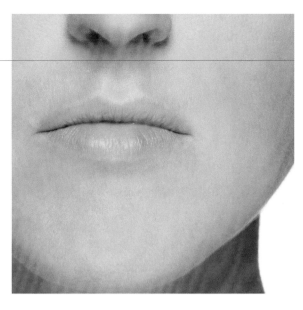

Choose a lip liner in a natural color that matches your lips—a brownish nude works well on most skin tones for correcting techniques like this. You don't want to thicken the lips, so don't work the liner around the bow, instead focus it on the outer part of the mouth, elongating and emphasizing the corners of the lips.

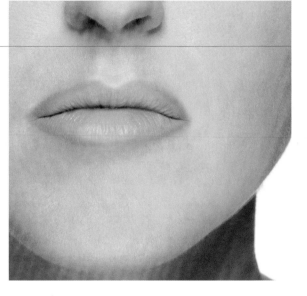

Once you have created a balanced shape at the outer corners, blend the lip liner out onto the whole lip to give a good base for the lipstick to adhere to. Use a creamy gloss stick with a slightly satiny finish in a soft brownish nude. Remember, it is best to steer clear of dark colors, as they will make your mouth look smaller.

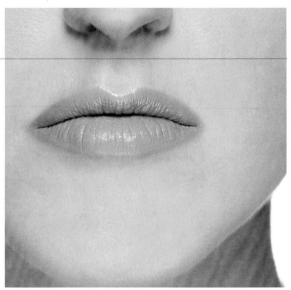

thin lips

Thin lips are a big concern for many women and the bad news is that lips get thinner as we grow older (see pages 184–7). Think of the golden rule: dark colors push things back, light colors bring them forward, so pale shades, glossy textures, and light-reflecting pigments will help to give the illusion of fuller lips. The big no-nos are dark colors and matte finishes.

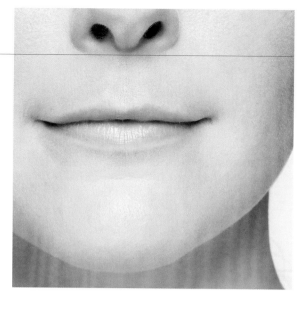

Choose a creamy lip pencil in a shade a little warmer than your skin tone. Starting with the bow, line the lips a mere fraction outside the natural lip line, focusing on deepening and thickening it. Be careful not to go onto the skin, as the lip liner will accentuate the fine hairs around your mouth. Bring the liner as far down to the corners of your mouth as you can without it looking artificial, and keep the emphasis on the bow and the middle of the bottom lip.

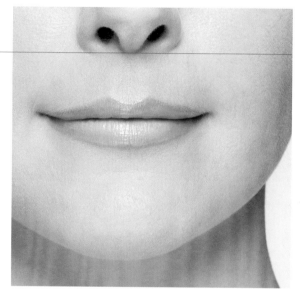

Apply a little cream highlighter above the bow, just outside the lip liner—this will catch the light and help to "lift" the lips. Apply a creamy lipstick to both lips. I chose a warm rose-pink glosstick from my range; it has a lovely sheen to it but with the creaminess of a rich lipstick. Lastly, add a dab of highlighter in the center of the bottom lip so the light catches it.

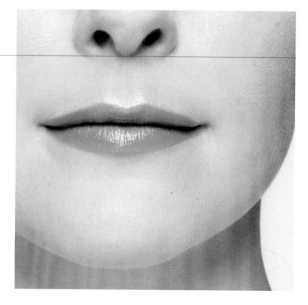

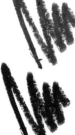
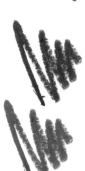

LIP LINER

You either love lip liner or you don't. But if you like wearing bold lipstick and want it to last longer, I urge you to give lip liner a try.

Lip liners shape and define the mouth, creating a smooth, even outline. They can be use to correct imperfections or asymmetry, prevent lipstick from bleeding at the edges, and, when used over the entire lip, keep lipstick in place for longer.

what to look for in a lip liner

TEXTURE Lip liners are normally wax-based. You don't want one that is too greasy, as you want the color to set quickly, and you don't want one that is so hard that it pulls on the lips as you apply it, so opt for a creamy wax texture.

COLOR For a nude look, pick the shade closest to your natural lip color or one shade warmer, but definitely no lighter. If you are going for a strong look, match the liner as closely as possible to your lipstick.

# #
How to apply lip liner

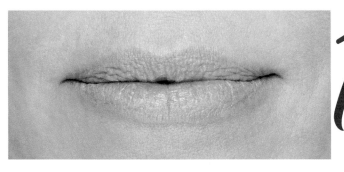

1 Prep the mouth using a lip primer, a dab of foundation, or a creamy concealer. This neutralizes the natural lip color so that you can achieve a really even, precise finish. Using my Lip Perfector just outside the lip line will ensure that you can create a really defined line with the lip liner.

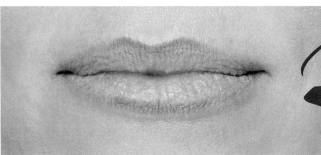

2 Start by outlining the bow, beginning at the center of the V and making sure both sides are exact mirror images of each other. Then balance the mouth by emphasizing the middle of the bottom lip, drawing either just inside or just outside the natural lip line if you need to correct the shape.

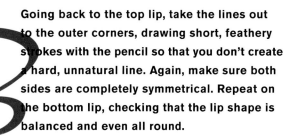

3 Going back to the top lip, take the lines out to the outer corners, drawing short, feathery strokes with the pencil so that you don't create a hard, unnatural line. Again, make sure both sides are completely symmetrical. Repeat on the bottom lip, checking that the lip shape is balanced and even all round.

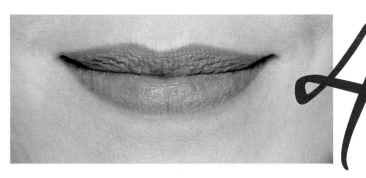

4 Fill in the rest of the lip with the pencil, creating an even base for the lipstick to adhere to and ensuring that it holds in place for longer. If you are using a strong color, go over the pencil with a brush to really work it into the creases in the lips for a smooth base. If your lipstick does wear off, you will still have an all-over color rather than just an outline.

PRO TRICK
Heat up the tip of the pencil by drawing over the back of your hand before applying it to your mouth.

LIP**STICK**

Whether you are a lover of nude lips, luscious gloss, sheer color, or rich red, lipstick provides an easy way to change your look, taking you from girl next door to sexy siren with just a swipe of color—it's an instant pick-me-up.

formulas and finishes

Choosing the right lipstick is not just down to picking a color that suits you (see page 98). There is also an array of formulas—long-lasting, plumping, hydrating, to name but a few—and finishes—stain, sheer, satin, creamy, gloss, matte, and metallic—to find your way around.

In my range the bestsellers are satin lipsticks, which are the most wearable and flattering for everyone. Neither too glossy nor too matte, a satin finish offers the best of everything. Here are some pointers to help you navigate your way around the beauty counter.

The main things to decide are:

What finish you want
sheer, creamy, matte, gloss

What formula you need
hydrating, long-lasting, plumping

What color suits you
from nudes through pinks and apricots to reds and browns

HELPFUL HINTS

\# Lipsticks combined with balms are a good option if you suffer from dry lips and can't live without your balm, as they provide the benefits of a moisturizer and SPF as well as the color, all in one bullet.

\# Hybrid lipsticks, such as the hydrating Glosssticks in my range, combine the creamy texture of a lipstick with a glossy finish. The colors are bright, but they contain less pigment, so they give a sheerer finish on the mouth than the equivalent lipstick. This means you can experiment with stronger, harder-to-wear colors.

\# Matte finishes are difficult to wear—they can be aging and make a small mouth seem smaller—so proceed with caution unless you have very full lips.

\# Silicone is drying, so look for silicone-free lipstick formulations.

\# Long-lasting formulas can be drying because of their high pigment content, so leave them for the evening when you will really benefit from them—when you are out eating and drinking, for example—and use tinted balm, gloss, or stain during the day.

\# My least favorite lipsticks are metallic— I prefer to use a highlighter just above the bow and in the center of the lower lip to lift the mouth.

\# Stains last a long time, but you shouldn't apply them on bare lips, as they are drying. Always use a balm underneath.

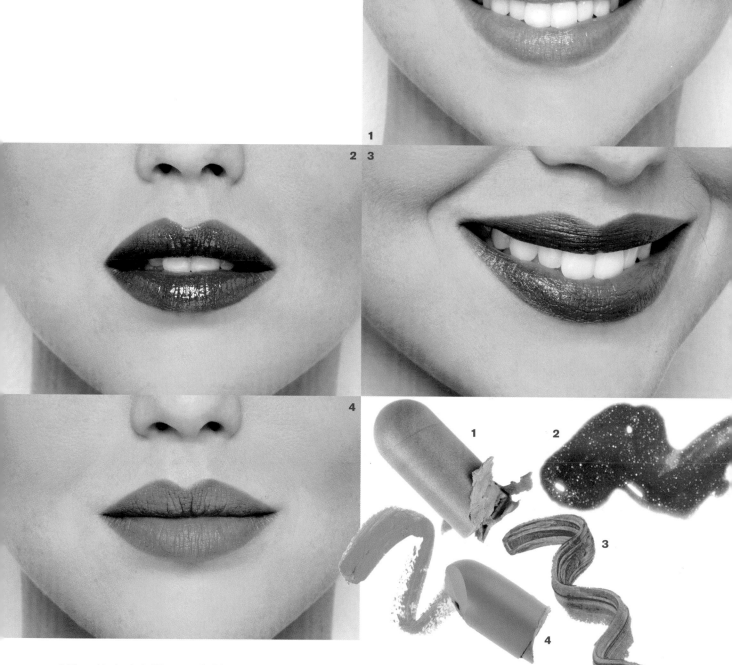

1 Tinted balm is brilliant for everyday, as it is easy to apply and easy to wear, offering all the benefits of its moisturizing, nourishing ingredients, while giving a natural hint of color to the lips.

2 Gloss is a lovely, flirty finish for the lips, giving them a luscious, sensual texture. Modern glosses aren't too sticky and can be worn on their own during the day or layered over a stain or lipstick for a more dramatic pout. It tends to come off quite quickly, so be prepared to reapply it regularly.

3 Satin lipstick gives a rich, creamy coverage with a slightly glossy finish. It looks good in all colors, and the slight sheen makes it flattering and wearable for everyone—an all-round bestseller.

4 Matte color makes a bold statement that looks stunning on fuller mouths, especially in classic Hollywood-starlet-red. Be careful if you are older, or if you have a small mouth or thin lips, as matte finishes can look harsh and aging.

colors
and tones

Most people gravitate naturally to the lipstick colors that suit them—you tend to know instinctively whether you are a pink person or an orange-brown person, for example.

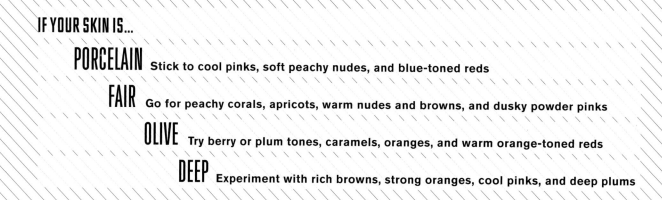

IF YOUR SKIN IS...

PORCELAIN Stick to cool pinks, soft peachy nudes, and blue-toned reds

FAIR Go for peachy corals, apricots, warm nudes and browns, and dusky powder pinks

OLIVE Try berry or plum tones, caramels, oranges, and warm orange-toned reds

DEEP Experiment with rich browns, strong oranges, cool pinks, and deep plums

GOLDEN RULES

Dark colors are generally harder to wear than paler shades. They can be more draining and aging, and you also need to be more accurate in your application, as any slips will be obvious.

Light and bright lipsticks will be more flattering if you have a small mouth or thin lips.

Never wear lipstick paler than your skin—it will make you look dead.

When you are wearing a dramatic, bold lipstick, keep the rest of your make-up minimal so that nothing competes for attention and you don't look overly made-up.

BERRY-STAINED LIPS

I love a bitten-lip look and there are a few ways to achieve it:

Dot a deep berry-colored lip liner all over your lips and blend it with your finger or a lip brush, so it looks really natural and subtle but is long-lasting.

Outline the lips with lip liner and then fill in the whole lip area. This gives a matte red-wine look that lasts a long time.

Use your finger as a tool: apply a berry-red lipstick to your forefinger and then push the color into your lips. This creates a stainlike finish.

If you are a red-lip girl, embrace it— don't just save it for a night out.

Most-wearable lip colors

Lipsticks can make or break a makeover, so getting the right shade is key. Everyone's skin tends to have a warmth or coolness to it: skin with yellow or orange undertones is described as warm, while skin with pink or red undertones is cool. Warm skin tends to suit colors with red or orange tones, while cool skin looks great in shades that have a blue tone to them.

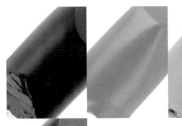

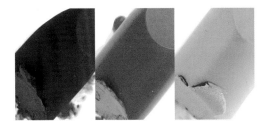

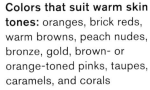

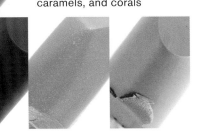

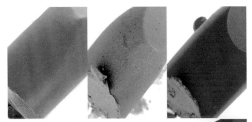

Colors that suit warm skin tones: oranges, brick reds, warm browns, peach nudes, bronze, gold, brown- or orange-toned pinks, taupes, caramels, and corals

Colors that suit cool skin tones: all pinks with a blue undertone, pink-based nudes, pink-based browns; nothing with orange tones

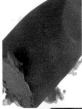

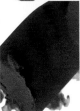

Colors that are wearable for everyone: wine shades, plum, peach, brownish pinks, mahogany, and poppy red—these colors have a mix of both cool and warm tones

HOW TO CHOOSE A COLOR

Don't rush—take as long as you need. If you can, try a lipstick on your lips to test the true color (use a Q-tip to apply it). Or, instead of trying it out on the back of your hand, which is not the same color as your mouth, try it on your fingertip, which is closer in color to your lips because of the concentration of blood vessels there, and hold it up to your mouth to see if it suits you. This will show you the true texture of the lipstick, too.

Go nude Nudes and natural brown tones are incredibly versatile, as they complement and blend with all skin tones. Always choose a shade that is warmer than your skin. We sell more lipsticks in the nude color range than reds and pinks—the bestseller is Audrey, a rich plummy-brown nude.

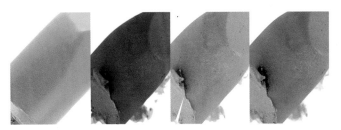

applying lipstick

Lipstick can, of course, be applied straight from the tube, which is ideal if you are out and about, but using a lip brush will give you more control and precision. It also results in a lighter coat of color than when you apply lipstick direct. As always, work in good light and take your time.

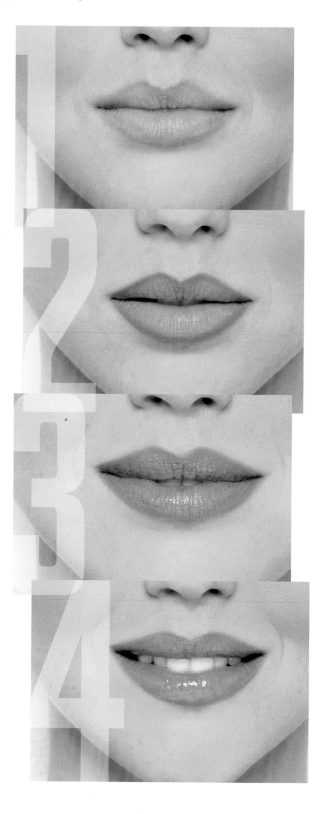

1 PRIME

Some people have high pigmentation in their lips, which can alter the color of the lipstick when it is applied to their mouth. Neutralize this using a priming product such as my Lip Perfector, or a little foundation or creamy concealer. The Lip Perfector is a pencil, so you can use it around the mouth to camouflage any sun damage and give you a really sharp, defined line when you apply lip liner. Use it like a primer over the surface of the lips, so the true color of the lipstick can come through.

2 LIP LINER

Choose a shade of lip liner that matches your skin or your lipstick. Starting in the center of the V, carefully outline the mouth, making sure both sides are symmetrical and the top and bottom lips are balanced (see page 95). Color in the surface of the mouth to provide a base for the lipstick and blend with a lip brush for a smooth and even coverage.

3 LIPSTICK

Using a lip brush, paint on the lipstick, working from the outside in and making sure the coverage is even. Use the tip of the brush for the edges and the flat of the brush to fill in larger areas. Blot with a tissue and then layer on another coat.

4 GLOSS

Use the wand to dab a little gloss onto your finger or the back of your hand (this avoids tainting your gloss with lipstick color). Then apply a little gloss on the top of the bow and the center of the bottom lip with your finger or the lip brush. The gloss will catch the light and make your lips look fuller.

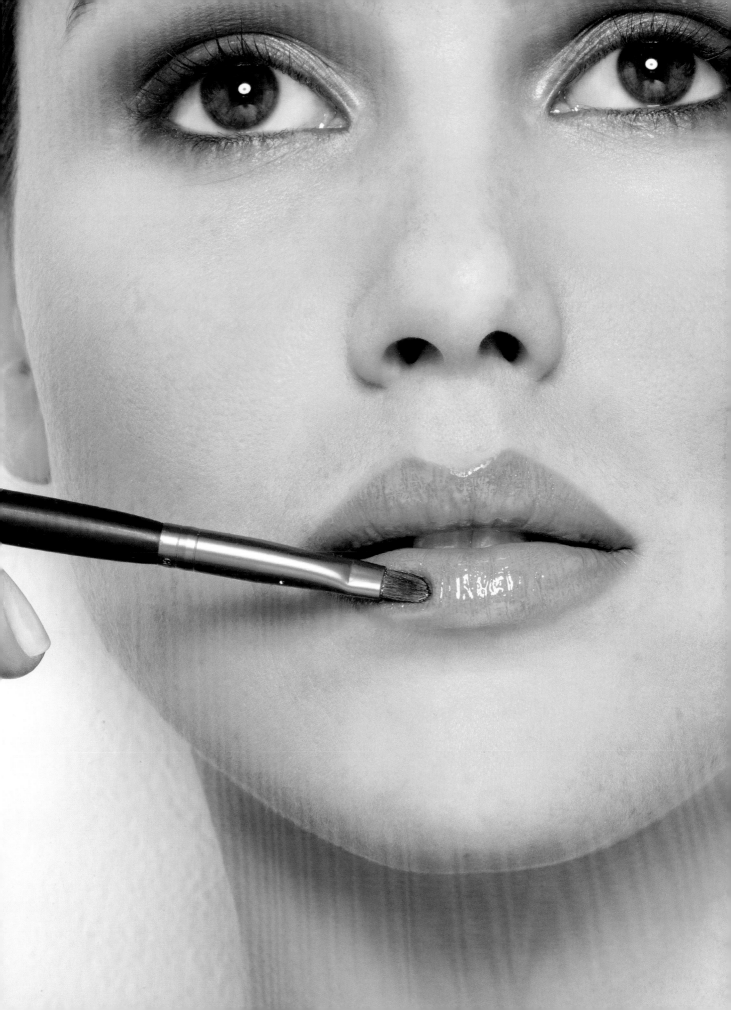

CLASSIC LIP AND CHEEK COLOR COMBINATIONS

Unless you are going for a statement look, lip and cheek colors should complement your skin and have similar undertones, so that nothing clashes or competes for attention.

for porcelain skin

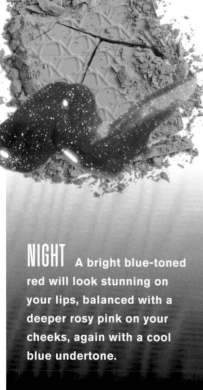

NIGHT A bright blue-toned red will look stunning on your lips, balanced with a deeper rosy pink on your cheeks, again with a cool blue undertone.

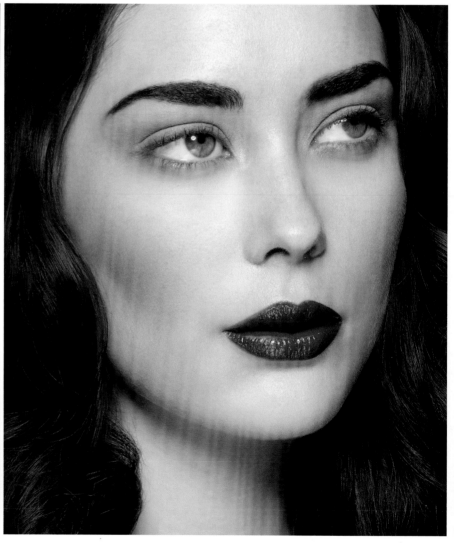

Above right Classic red gloss layered over a matching lip pencil, with cheeks subtly warmed with a pinky beige blush, is stunning on porcelain skin for the evening.

★ TOP TIPS

\# Look for soft pink and beige colors with cool undertones, such as sandy pink and pale baby pink.

\# Pair soft, cool pink cheeks with nude lips.

\# Stay away from anything with orange or warm golden tones.

DAY The pale lip and cheek colors that work best on you for a soft, natural look may seem almost too light when they are in the palette, but you only need to go a couple of shades deeper than your alabaster skin to give you a fresh glow.

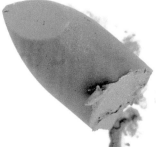

Above Stronger cheek colors can be applied sparingly for a pretty day look and cream blush blends to a light, natural finish. The pink-nude lipstick tones beautifully.

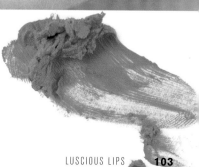

DAY Soft peach or powdery, dusky pinks are flattering on fair skin, and any of the brownish "dirty" pinks work well for a nude daytime look.

for fair skin

NIGHT For a stronger nighttime look, go for a warm red, a pinky red, or an apricot red, depending on how warm or cool your skin is. Choose a deeper blush than for daytime, making sure it tones with your lipstick, so they don't clash.

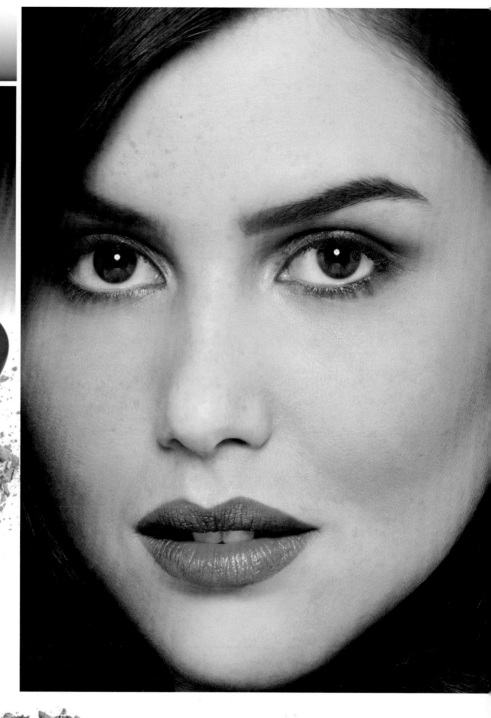

Right Soft pink powder blush can be gradually built up in intensity to balance a stronger berry lipstick that gives a cool-toned pink satin finish.

Opposite Creamy hydrating lipstick in a light rose pink combines with a soft pearl bronzing trio for a subtle naturally warm look.

★ TOP TIPS

\# You can wear any of the neutral colors, such as warm pinks and dusty rose.

\# Pale beige is perfect for shading, giving subtle results on fair skin.

\# Soft, pale apricot shades can work well on fair skin, as long as it doesn't have very cool (pink) undertones.

for olive skin

DAY Warm orange-toned peach and light apricot shades work well for a daytime look when you have a yellow undertone to your skin. If you have a deeper orange undertone, you can go for a much richer red-toned apricot or coral. For a nude lip, go for a warm brown shade or a light coral gloss.

Right Soft orange tones on both cheeks and lips are really flattering for olive skin. A cream blush and a light glossy lipstick are complementary textures.

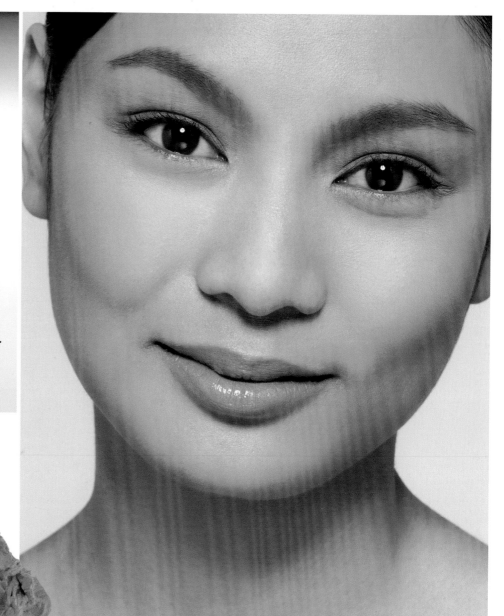

Opposite Rich red lipstick needs a deeper cheek color for the evening. A bronze and pink powder duo can be blended together or either side can be used separately.

⭐ TOP TIPS

\# Warm red-toned apricots work well on olive skin—the more tan your skin, the deeper you can go, but stick to the softer peachier shades if your skin is pale olive.

\# Orangy gold colors suit deep olive or tan skin.

\# Coral blush looks stunning if you have warm (yellow-toned) or Asian skin.

NIGHT For the evening, a deep berry lip color that has some warmth to it pairs well with a rich, warm apricot blush.

for deep skin

DAY For a natural look, you just need to warm up the skin a little, depending on its depth and tone. If you have warm skin, go for golden hues for a daytime look. If your skin has cool undertones, blue-based pinks will enhance it.

Above Coral gloss and pink-apricot blush are a pretty combination for a daytime look, matching the warm skin tones perfectly.

⭐ TOP TIPS

For day, look for corals, apricots, and pinky red pomegranate tones.

Deep rich reds, such as raison, berry, and plum, look stunning on your lips for a dramatic look.

Warm chocolaty browns are very flattering.

Above Liquid stain can be used on both the cheeks and lips for a sheer natural finish that can be built up in intensity. For extra glamour, apply a plum lipstick with a dab of clear gloss to catch the light.

NIGHT
Rich berry-reds give you glamorous lips. Pair them with a deep plum or pomegranate blush.

The 10 most-asked questions about lips

1

What shade of red can I wear?

Poppy red and wine-colored reds suit most women. As a general guide, if you have pink-toned or very pale, porcelain skin, cool blue-based reds will look good on you; if you have a warmer complexion with yellow or orange undertones, choose orange-based reds; if you have dark skin, go for rich plum or berry red.

2

How can I make my lipstick last longer?

Prep and prime your lips well to create a good canvas to work on—use a lip primer such as my Lip Perfector, or a dab of foundation or concealer. After outlining your lips, apply lip liner over the whole surface to provide a smooth, even undercoat of color and a waxy base for the lipstick to adhere to. Apply one coat of lipstick, then blot it with a tissue and layer on another coat. For a matte finish, a dusting of translucent powder or blush patted on top of the lipstick will give it excellent staying power.

3

How can I stop my lipstick from "bleeding?"

This is when a lipstick or gloss migrates beyond the lip line—oily lipsticks and liquid glosses and stains travel more, so choose thicker, drier, and less greasy formulas. Prep your lips well before outlining them with a waxy lip liner that will help to create a barrier to hold the lipstick in place. Spend time working it into any fine lines along the lip line. Use a lip brush to apply a little translucent powder around the edges of the mouth—not on the lips—to set it. (See page 180.)

4

How can I make my lips look bigger?

Use a lip liner in a color that matches your lips (for a nude look) or your lipstick (for a bolder look) and outline your lips just a fraction outside your natural lip line (see page 93). Choose paler colors in light-reflecting finishes and stay away from dark shades and matte textures, which make lips look smaller. Add a touch of gloss or highlighter to the center of the bottom lip and the top of the bow to catch and bounce the light. Plumping formulas can also help to make lips look fuller.

5

What lip color suits me best?

The key thing is to assess the undertones of your skin and work out whether your coloring is warm or cool. If you have warm (yellow-toned) skin, choose colors in the orange spectrum—anything from warm nudes and browns to peaches, apricots, corals, orange- or red-based pinks, and deeper orangy reds. If you have cool (pink-toned) skin, go for blue-toned pinks and reds and stay away from orange-based colors. Pink-based nudes and browns and deeper earthy browns all work well on cooler skin. How dark a color you can wear may be influenced by the depth of your skin tone and hair color—also take into consideration your age and the size of your lips. Remember, the natural pigment of your lips will influence the color of the lipstick, so if you can't try out a new color on your lips, try it on the pad of your finger and hold that up to your mouth to see how it suits you. (See pages 98–9.)

6

How can I increase the intensity of my lip color?

For a multilayered effect, apply your lipstick, then use a thick pencil to draw a series of vertical lines on your lips. Apply a second coat of lipstick and top it off with a final swipe of pencil to keep it all in place. This will achieve excellent hold, deep color, and the illusion of fuller lips.

7

Is there anything I can do if I don't like the color?

If you buy a shade that turns out to be too dark, bright, or pale for you, blend it with another lipstick or gloss to achieve a bespoke color that suits you perfectly.

8

What if my lipstick is too dark for me?

Turn it into a stain by blotting most of the lipstick off your lips for a subtle and long-lasting finish.

9

How can I stop my lipstick from drying out my lips?

Wear moisturizing balm underneath your lipstick. Most of the time when applying make-up the lips are left until last, so coat your lips in balm while you are doing the rest of your make-up. This will soften and condition them, ready for you to apply your lipstick.

10

How can I prevent my lip pencil from breaking

Put lip pencils in the icebox before you sharpen them—this makes the tips less likely to break off and gives a cleaner, sharper point. Warm up the tip by drawing on the back of your hand before lining your lips.

fashion make-up

The worlds of fashion and cosmetics are inextricably intertwined, with the make-up themes seen on the runways every season filtering down to main street, and the colors and textures showcased in all the major collections finding their way onto beauty counters everywhere.

I love fashion. It's part of me and is often what inspires me to bring out new colors—whether as an eyeliner, eyeshadow, lipstick, or gloss. The JK range that I produce is my runway-diffusion brand, which takes its lead from high-fashion make-up trends and makes them accessible to everyone. Fashion should be fun, and I like to encourage women to experiment and have fun with make-up, too.

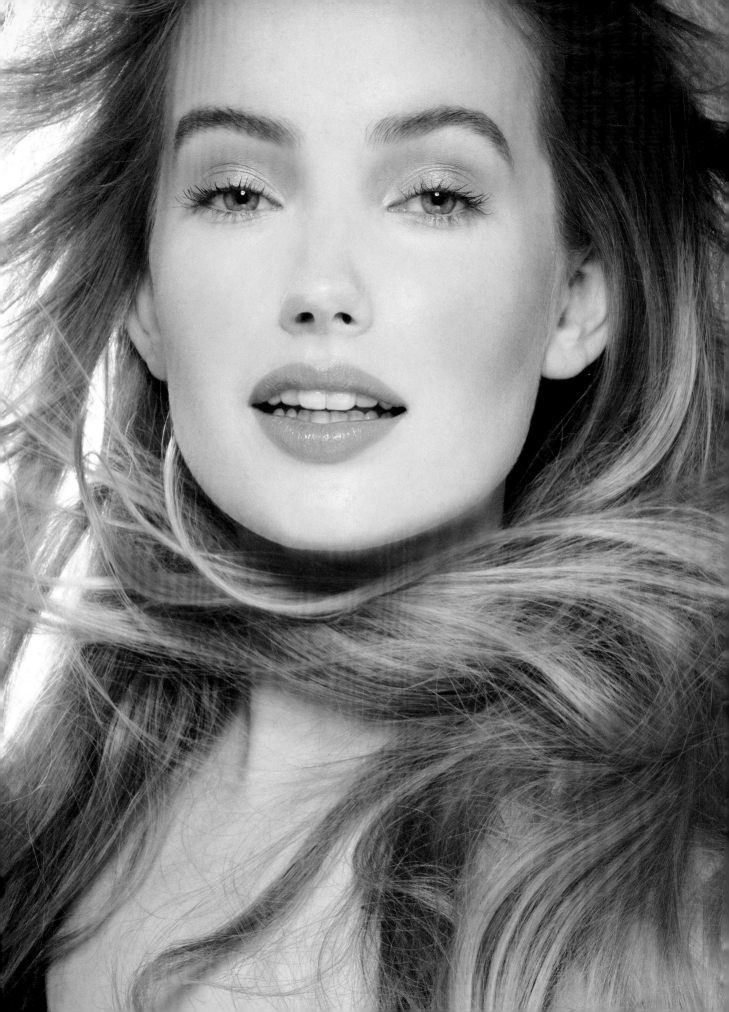

HOW TO WEAR COLOR

High-fashion looks, though inspiring, are mostly too extreme for everyday, so I wanted to interpret them in a wearable way. I used the same hot pink on the lips, eyes, and cheeks, to show how bold color can be used as a statement on different features.

the bold lip **The lips are where most women feel comfortable wearing the brightest colors. It is probably the "safest" way to go bold. The rest of the face must be flawless, with minimal make-up in neutral tones so that the statement color really stands out.**

Keep the eyes natural, with neat brows, a simple colorwash of soft pearl taupe eyeshadow (1) and black mascara (2). Use a "noncolor" blush (3)—similar to the skin tone but just a bit warmer—to give a little definition and structure to the cheeks.

To get a really sharp line and strong color, make sure the lip surface is perfect, without any flaky skin. Exfoliate the mouth, moisturize with a waxy balm, and then blot with a tissue to get rid of any greasiness (see pages 88–9).

Use a bright pink lip liner (4) to draw a perfectly symmetrical outline and then fill in the whole lip area (see page 95). Layer matching lipstick (5) on top, using a lip brush for precision.

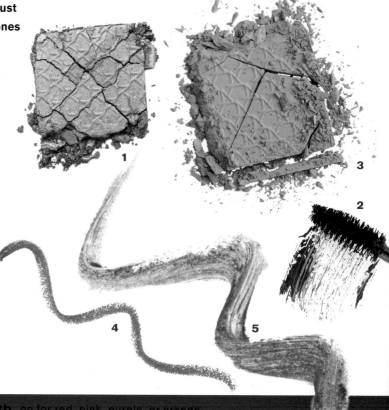

THE MOST WEARABLE BRIGHTS On the mouth, go for red, pink, purple, or orange.

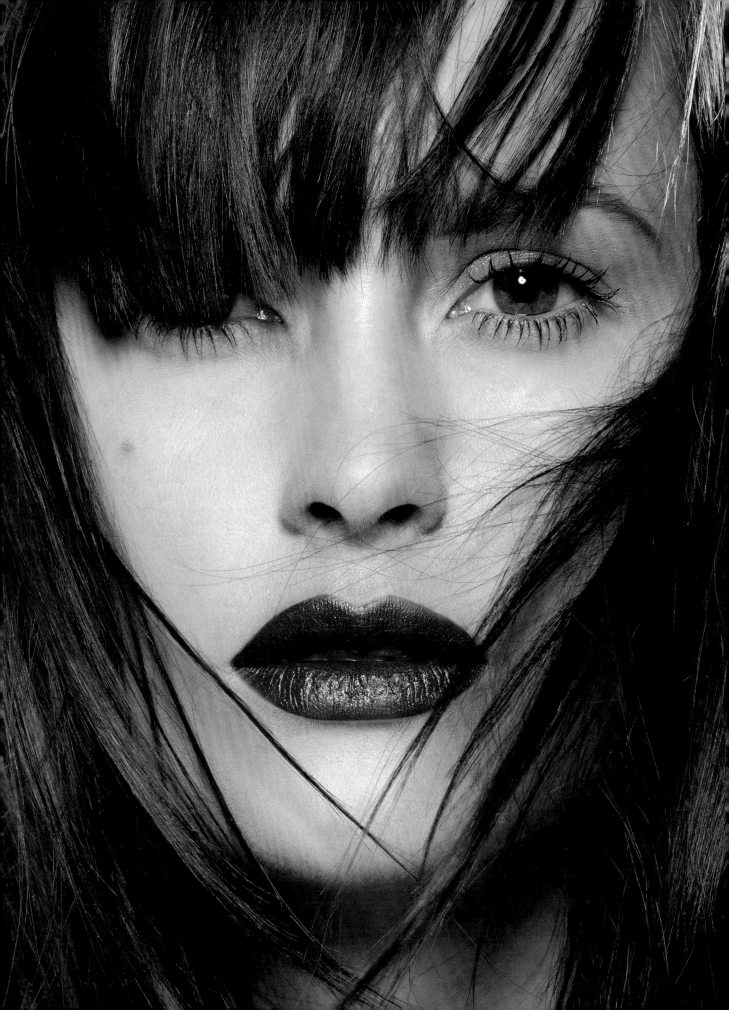

the bold eye

When you are wearing a bold color on the eyes, keep the rest of the face quite clean and plain but make a really sharp brow. I think a wash of just one bright color over the mobile lid and blended out looks gorgeous. You can mix two colors, but any more tends to look untidy.

Bold is beautiful, but bold make-up is for the brave and you need confidence to pull it off.

BOLD COLOR TRENDS THAT ANYONE CAN WEAR

Hot pinks and bold blues look amazing on the eyes, whatever your skin tone.

Fuchsia lips are one of the most wearable ways to go bold. The color works on everyone, as long as you don't blush easily or have strong red undertones.

Bright red lips are classic—choose a tomato red with more orange in it if you have warm skin and a cherry red with blue undertones if you have cool skin.

Define the brows with a natural pencil or powder. Work black eyeliner into the roots of the lashes (1) to give a good foundation for the color and create a sharp line.

Base the mobile lid with bright pink cream eyeshadow (2) and then layer the same color powder (3) on top. The cream creates a good base for blending and holds and intensifies the pigment. Blend the powder up above the socket, so you can see the color when the eye is open. You want a really soft finish that is completely even with no blotches or hard edges.

Apply two coats of black mascara (4).

Nothing should take away from the bold eyes, so just warm up the cheeks and give them a little definition with matte bronzer (5). Keep the lips natural and nude with a creamy lipstick (6).

THE MOST WEARABLE BRIGHTS On the eyes, try bright blue, aqua, pink, purple, citrus yellow, green, or orange.

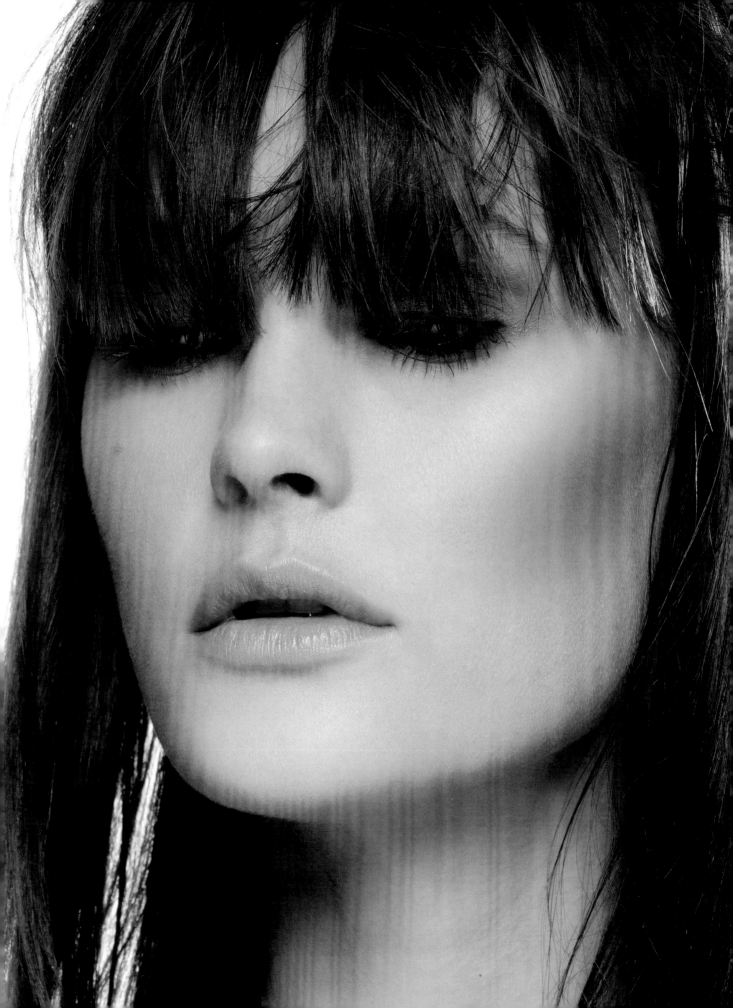

the bold cheek

If you are going to use a bright color on the face, the skin has to be completely uniform in color before you begin. Not one blemish or capillary should be seen. This dramatic cheek was created by just layering and layering powdered blush, to achieve the full intensity of the color with the softness of the powder finish. Use a brush smaller than a normal blush brush to give you sufficient control to keep the color on the cheekbones with the softness on the apples and up into the hairline.

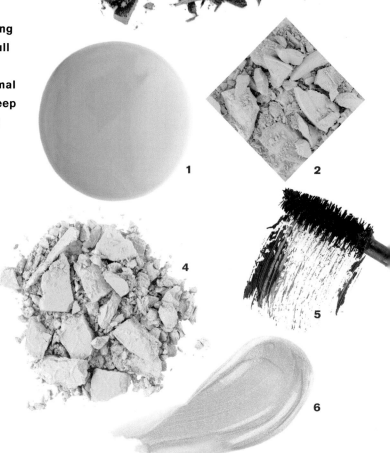

Natural is safe and pretty, but sometimes it's fun to stand out from the crowd.

GOLDEN RULES

Go bold on one part of the face only—lips, eyes, or cheeks. Whatever feature you want to draw attention to is where the bold color should be. If you've got a great mouth, why not show it off? If you've got fabulous cheekbones, focus on those.

If you want a bold color to really stand out, it has to slightly clash with your skin tone, not blend with it.

When working with bold colors, choose high-pigment products so you don't have to use too much.

Apply full-coverage foundation (1) to hide any pigmentation on the skin. Then powder (2) the area that you are going to blush—along the cheekbones and into the hollows—because that helps the color to blend very softly: if there is any oiliness on the skin, it will be blotchy.

Apply bright pink powder blush (3) near the top of the cheekbones and blend, blend, blend with small circular movements. Keep layering and blending until the color is the intensity you want.

Brush a soft pearl camel eyeshadow (4) over the eyelids and then apply black mascara (5). Coat the lips with a sheer pink nude gloss (6).

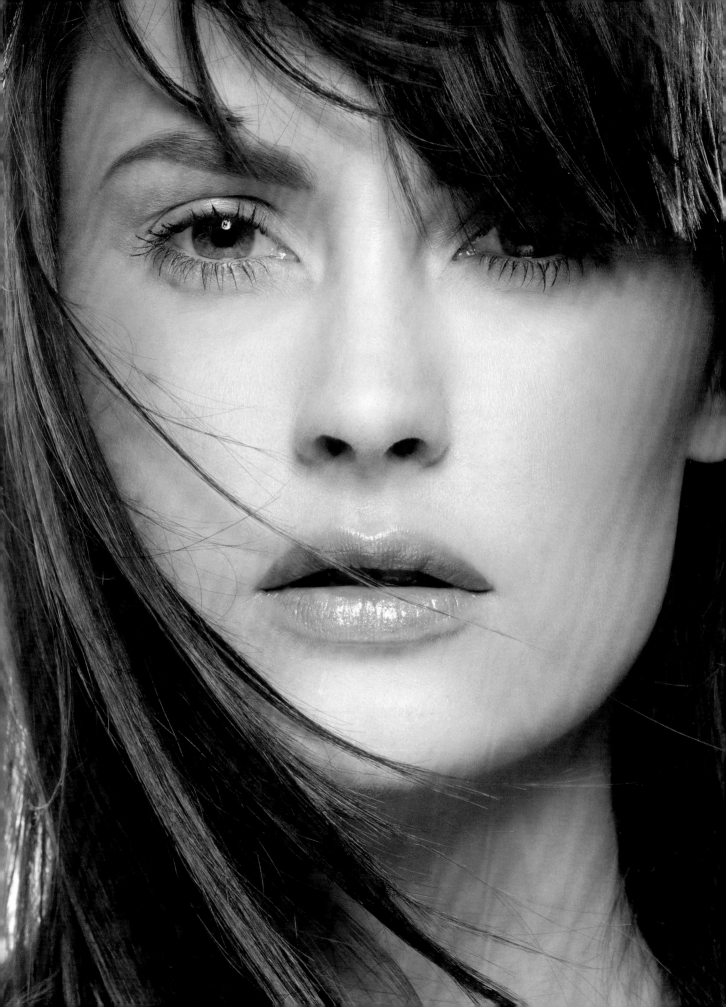

KEY RUNWAY
TRENDS

There are certain classic fashion looks that are rarely out of style. Key trends, such as florals, neon, nudes, and monochrome, come around on the fashion carousel time after time. The nuances may shift with new interpretations, but the basic ethos remains the same.

floral

Whether ditsy and cute, painterly and romantic, or bright and splashy, florals nearly always feature in Spring/Summer collections. The look is feminine, romantic, and pretty—think long, floaty chiffon and relaxed, natural hair. The make-up is soft, wearable, and flattering, with an emphasis on all shades of pink and peach, pretty pastel hues, and pearl or shimmer textures. The skin looks dewy and healthy, and all the colors are softly blended. I decided to make a statement on the mouth with a strong but really pretty shade of pink, but a softer pink or a peachy shade would also work well.

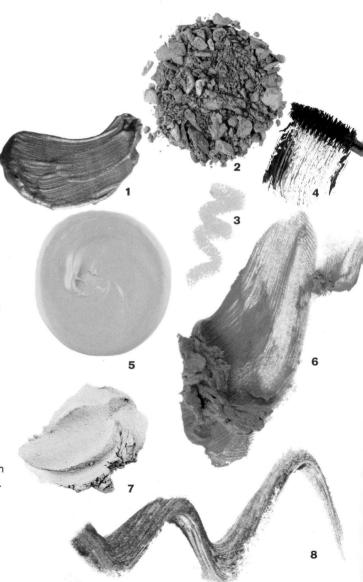

Eyes Brush up the brows and use a natural powder for that full, youthful look. Apply a natural warm taupe eye cream (1) over the mobile lid, then layer a shimmery eyeshadow in the same color (2) on top. Blend it well, taking the color softly above the socket crease. Use a nude pencil (3) along the inner rims of the eyes to brighten them and apply black mascara (4).

Skin Even out the skin tone with tinted moisturizer (5) for a natural, dewy finish. Warm up the cheeks with a peach cream blush applied just under the cheekbones (6). Blend cream highlighter (7) along the cheekbones for extra radiance.

Lips Apply satin finish fuchsia lipstick (8) with a lip brush, keeping the shape soft and natural.

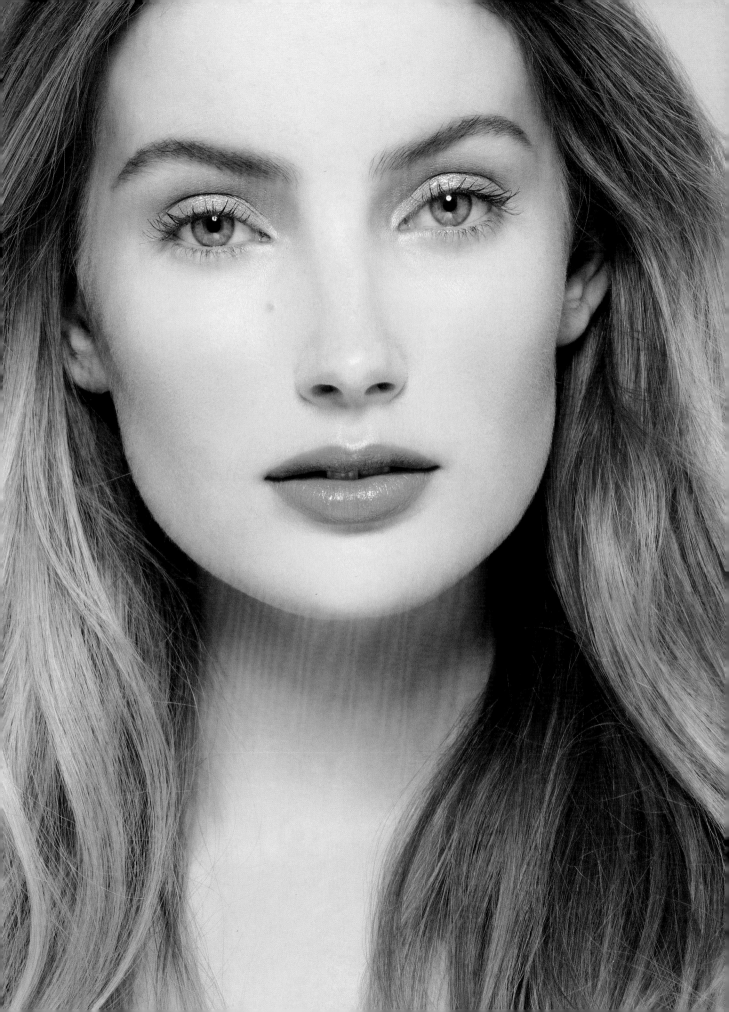

neon

Bold brights, color blocking, and eye-popping neons are often at the foundation of designers' retro- and, conversely, futuristic-inspired collections.

Interpreted in make-up, the neon trend is a harder one to wear away from the runway or fashion editorials. But, when done well, it is a perfect statement look for parties or festivals. The eyes are the easiest place to wear neons, and this stunning green eyeliner is really flattering against thick black lashes when the rest of the make-up is kept low-key.

EXTREME WAYS TO WEAR NEON

\# Block designs on the eyes make a bold statement—neon doesn't work if it is soft and blended.

\# Neon pink or orange work best on the lips—yellow can look stunning but extreme. Achieve this using a sheer lipstick with neon pigment pressed on top.

Eyes Brush up the brows and use a matching brow powder to make them look natural and full. Prime the lids to conceal any redness, and brighten the inner rims with a nude eye pencil (1). Work black pencil eyeliner (2) along the upper lash line and between the roots of the lashes to darken them and frame the neon. Using neon-green eyeliner (3) and a steady hand, paint a sharp line along the base of the lid from the inner corner to the outer corner, then flick it up the line of elevation (see page 45). Apply black mascara (4) and false lashes (5) to dramatize the eyes and ground the neon.

Skin Use medium-coverage foundation (6) and concealer to make sure the skin tone is even with no dark undereye circles. Powder the T-zone lightly to mattify the skin (7) and then warm up the cheeks with peachy blush (8).

Lips Keep the lips natural with a coat of pinky nude lipstick (9).

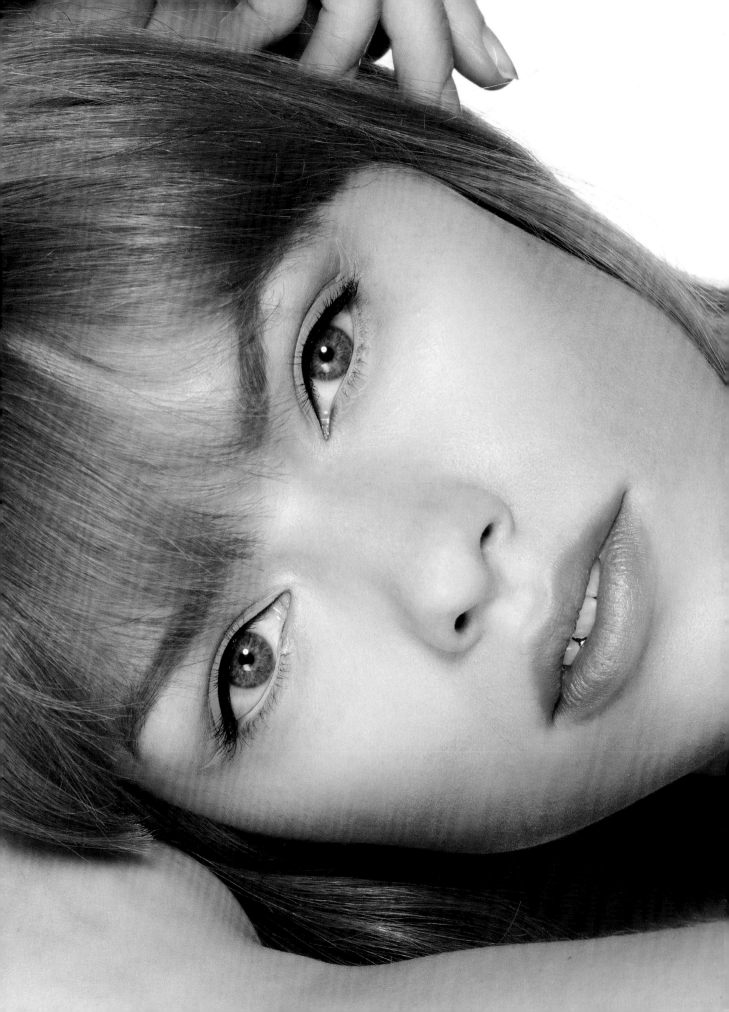

nude

The nude fashion trend is all about texture and drape—whether lace, silk, tailoring, chunky knits, or the finest cashmere—in muted neutrals, including taupe, gray, mink, cream, sand, and the palest pink and apricot. Barely-there make-up is a favorite for the runway, as it makes the models look amazing but doesn't steal the limelight from the clothes. Off the runway, it is also very flattering and wearable; it's what most women gravitate to for an everyday look. Nothing is a statement in the "no make-up make-up" look. You are simply using the warm, natural, earthy tones, which all blend together, to contour and shape the face.

KEY FEATURES OF "STEALTH" MAKE-UP

\# With nude make-up, the brows need to be strong and perfectly shaped to give the face structure.

\# The skin must be flawless but natural—you need to conceal blemishes or redness, but only apply foundation and concealer where you really need it.

\# Focus on enhancing your features subtly, without making a statement—all the colors should blend and tone together.

\# Take your time to blend everything really well for the most natural finish.

Eyes Darken the eyebrows and define the arch with a brow pencil (1). Apply eye primer (2) to the lids to create a smooth base and neutralize redness. Brush soft gold eyeshadow (3) over the mobile lids and work a deeper toning color (4) into the socket crease, blending it up and out. Work a black pencil eyeliner (5) between the roots of the lashes to darken and thicken them, then apply black mascara (6) and add corner lashes (7) to open and elongate the eyes.

Skin Apply foundation (8) and concealer where necessary to even out the skin tone. Contour the cheeks by blending soft apricot blush (9) into the hollows under the cheekbones and taking it out into the hairline to give the face definition. Add a touch of highlighter (10) along the outer part of the cheekbones and the browbones.

Lips A hybrid balm-lipstick duo in a pinky nude (11) keeps the lips moisturized and natural.

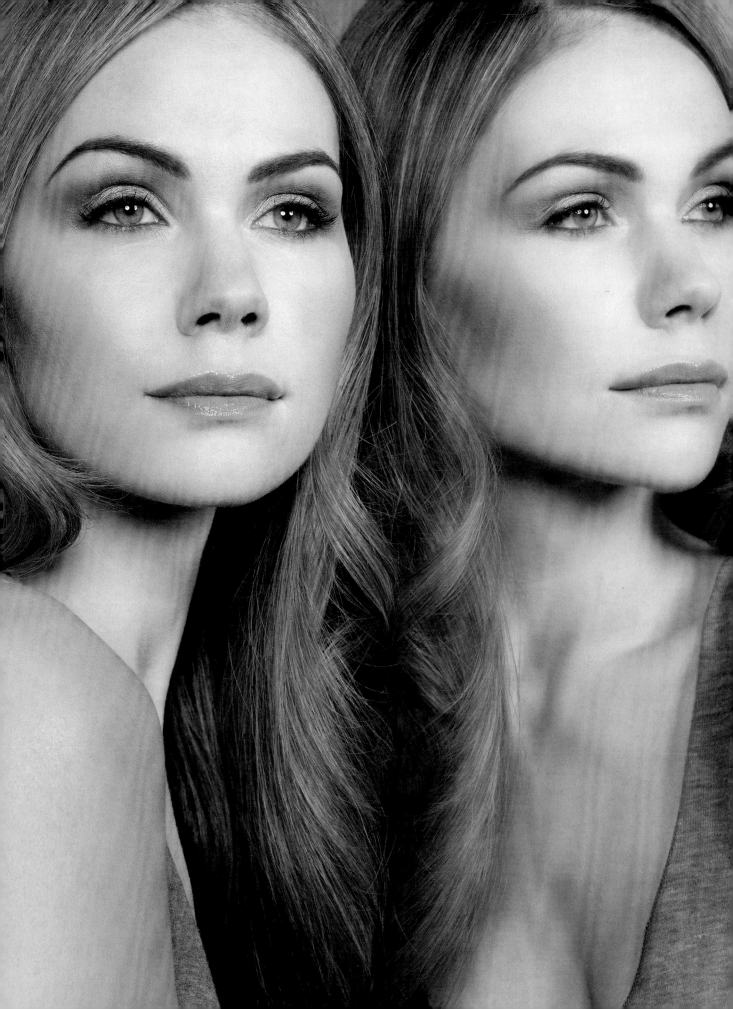

monochrome

The graphic monochrome look is synonymous with the 1960s, a decade that still influences contemporary fashion trends.

This is a strong, matte look that requires a certain level of skill to execute. Working with black and white is difficult, as you have to be much more precise than with colors that can be blended—so no shaky hands. When done right, the contrast between the strong eyes and the pale, matte face and lips can be very flattering.

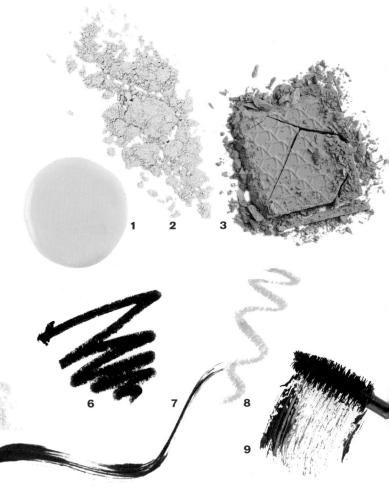

TOP TIPS FOR MONOCHROME MAKE-UP

\# Lighten and mattify the entire face before you do the eyes, as the skin needs to be as pale as it can be without looking ashy and artificial.

\# The eyebrows need to be as sharp, strong, and neat as the liner—an unkempt or natural brow won't look right with this look.

Skin Apply primer over the face and eyelids, followed by full-coverage foundation (1). Mattify the face with translucent powder (2), then brush a little nude, almost putty-colored blush (3) into the hollows of the cheeks to give the face definition and depth.

Eyes Use as dark a brow pencil as you can for your coloring (4) to deepen the color of the eyebrows and create a sharp shape, tapering the outer corners to a fine point. Brush a pale bone matte eyeshadow (5) over the eyelids. Work black pencil eyeliner (6) into the roots of the lashes and blend it along the lash lines.

Take a liquid or gel liner (7) and work on the top lid first. Draw from the inner corner along the lash line to the outer corner, then take the line out horizontally toward your ear. Taper the line out from the inner corner, so it is thicker on the outer third of the eye, and join it up with the end of the horizontal line at the outer corner to create an arrowhead shape.

On the lower lash line, dot the liner from the center of the eye to level with the end of the upper horizontal line. Join the dots to make a straight line parallel to the one above. Join the lines at the outer corner of the eye so that it is completely outlined.

Use a nude pencil (8) along the inner rims to open up the eyes, and then apply black mascara (9).

Lips Keep the lips completely nude and pale, using just a lip primer (10) to conceal the natural redness.

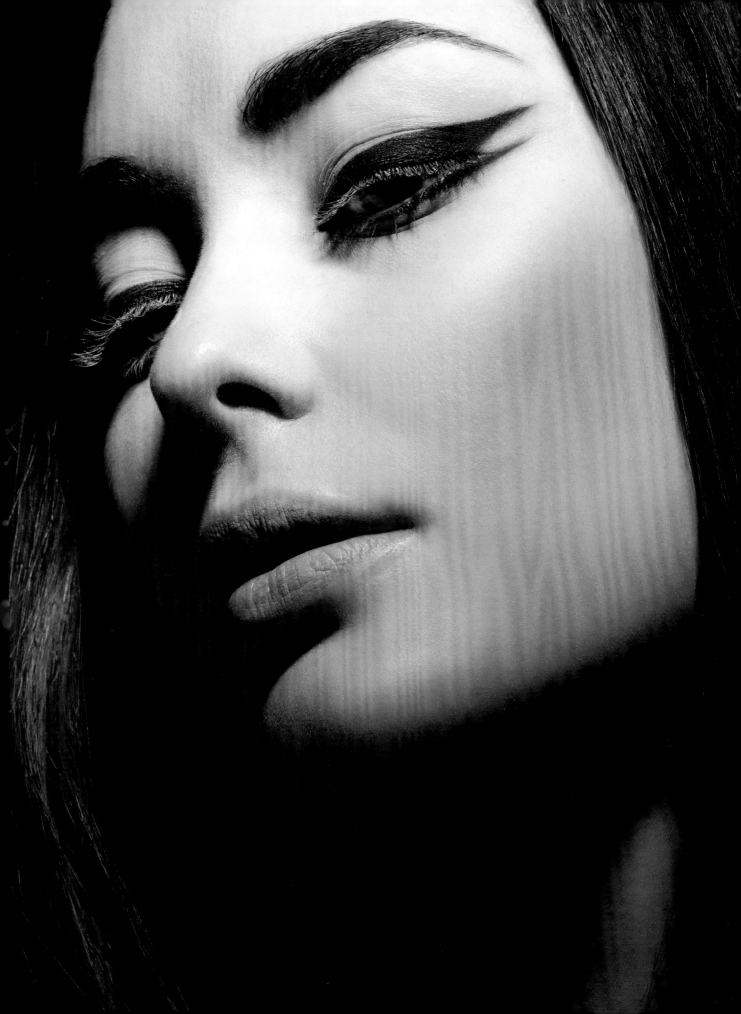

the *timeless* look

There are certain make-up looks that aren't subject to the vagaries of fashion. Synonymous with some of the most beautiful women of all time, these elegant, wearable looks are pure classics that will never go out of style.

In the years following the Second World War, the Hollywood stars of the Silver Screen were the beauty icons to which women aspired. Supremely alluring and always immaculate, timeless beauties such as Grace Kelly, Audrey Hepburn, and Sophia Loren were—and still are—the epitome of femininity, sophistication, and glamour.

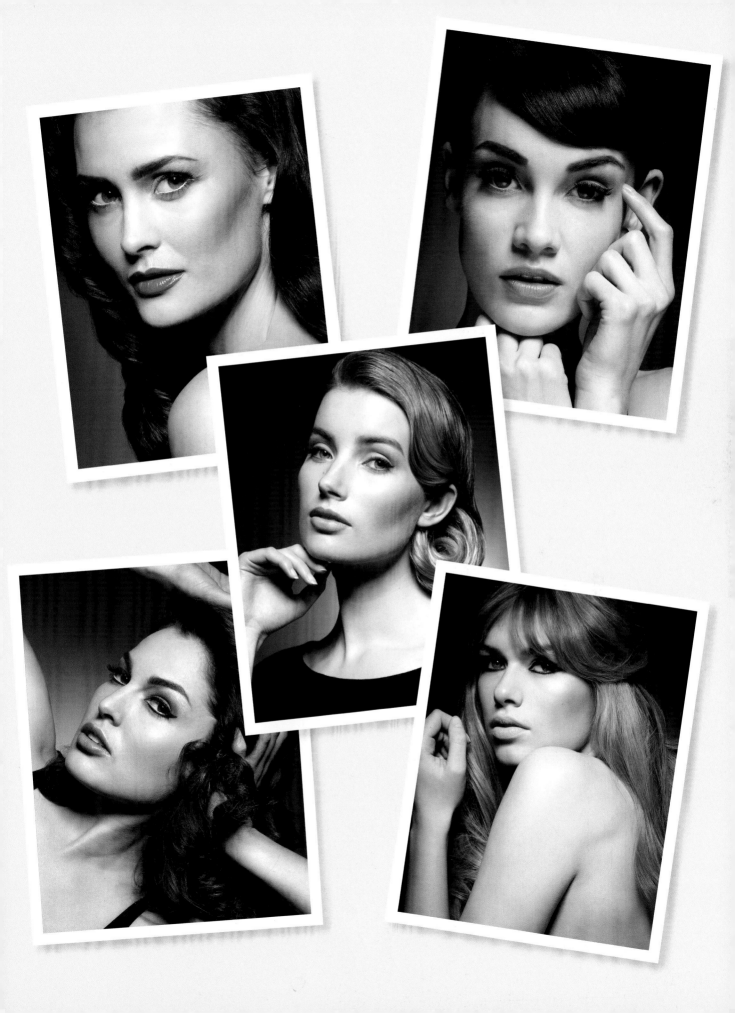

timeless look of

Brigitte Bardot

French former model and actress Brigitte Bardot is one of the quintessential sex symbols of the late 1950s and early 1960s, known for her smoky bedroom eyes, soft nude pout, and tousled blonde hair. Her signature make-up is all about the dramatic eyes accentuated with heavy, smudged eyeliner and long, thick lashes, paired with pale apricot lips that were sometimes matte, sometimes glossy. Her skin was flawless and fresh, with sculpted cheekbones accented with soft peachy pink blush or lightly bronzed for a sunkissed look.

Bardot's kohl-rimmed eyes, heavy lashes, and pale lips are copied time and again. It's the ultimate sex-kitten look

KEYNOTES OF THE BRIGITTE BARDOT LOOK

Keep the colors of all your make-up very neutral.
Focus on emphasizing the eyes, with heavy eyeliner applied all the way around the rims.
Thick mascara and false lashes help to create that trademark heavy-lidded flutter.
Skin must be flawless and pale with a luminous, almost dewy finish, so use tinted moisturizer or light liquid foundation and a dusting of light-reflecting powder if you need it.
Sculpt the cheeks using peachy pink blush and apply highlighter along the cheekbones to accentuate them.
Keep the lips neutral and matte so the eyes really stand out.

Top tip Classic smoky eyes (see pages 72–5) work really well for a more dramatic nighttime version of this look. Apply gray eyeshadow from the lash line to the crease and blend it out with small circular motions.

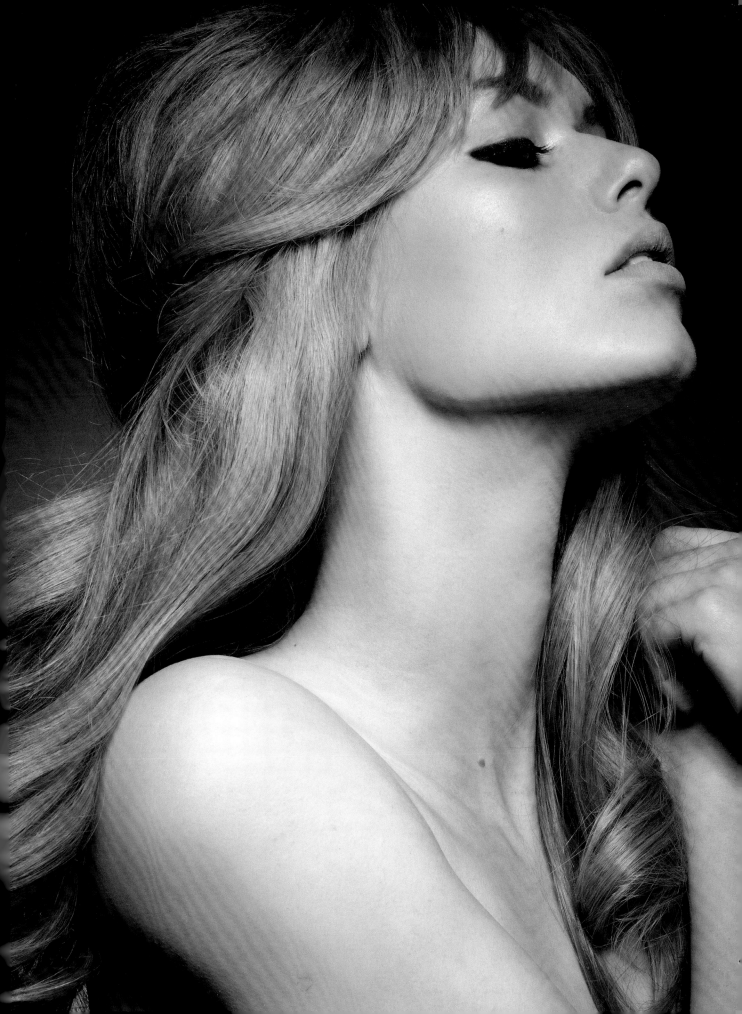

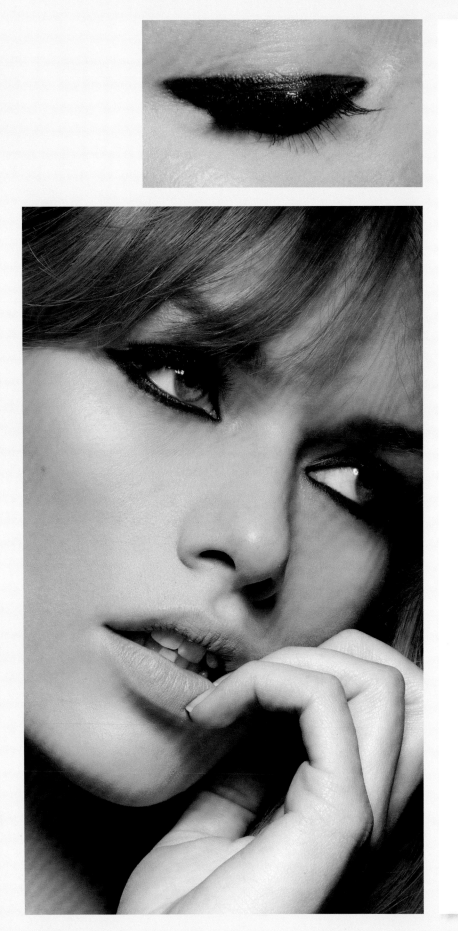

EYES Sultry kohl-rimmed eyes and heavy lashes

1 Go over the eyebrows with matching brow powder to create natural fullness.

2 Prime the eyelid to provide a smooth base and neutralize any redness.

3 Blend a nude powder eyeshadow over the entire lid.

4 Using a black pencil eyeliner, draw along the upper and lower lash lines, joining up at the inner and outer corners so the eyes are fully encircled. Then fill in the waterlines.

5 Use a liner brush to go around the rim of the eyes with black wet/dry powder liner for a soft, smudged effect.

6 Apply lots of lengthening, thickening mascara to the top and bottom lashes. Then add false lashes for extra drama.

SKIN Dewy radiant skin

7 Prep the skin with a primer to create a smooth hydrated base, then even out the skin tone using a sheer tinted moisturizer. Use concealer if you need to cover any imperfections.

8 Apply a little peach cream blush to the apples of your cheek to create a sheer warm flush.

9 Blend a little highlighter onto the high points of your face to make the skin look dewy and fresh.

LIPS Nude matte lips

10 Make sure the lips are exfoliated and moisturized. Then either brush a small amount of foundation onto your lips to create a nude matte finish or apply a pale nude lipstick and mattify it with powder.

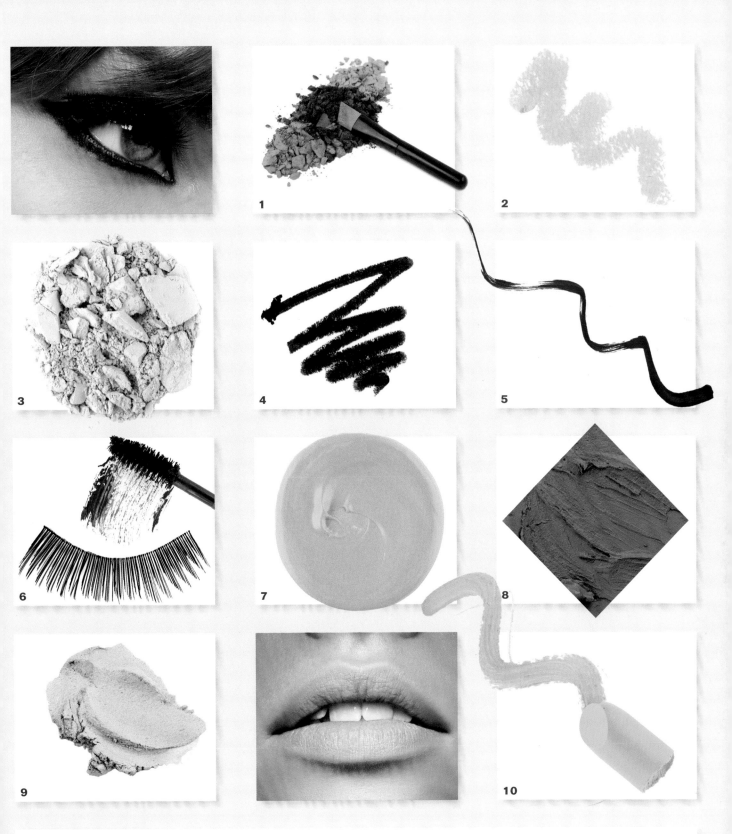

VARIATIONS ON A THEME

\# As an alternative to matte lips, use a tinted lip balm or light gloss in soft pink or apricot.

\# If your skin isn't naturally pale, embrace the sunkissed version of this look by using a soft pearl bronzer to sculpt your cheeks, with a gold-toned highlighter on the cheekbones.

timeless look of

Audrey Hepburn

As ingénue Holly Golightly in 1961's *Breakfast at Tiffany's*, Audrey Hepburn inspired a style that everyone wanted to copy. Her large wide-open eyes were indisputably the focus of her face, with thick liquid liner along the upper lash lines that flicked up toward the end of the eyebrows, which were strong with a pronounced arch. She peered out innocently from under the long, curled lashes that fluttered alluringly. Her cheeks were naturally flushed and her lips were kept light in soft pinks or nudes.

Audrey's look epitomizes youthful innocence. All the drama is on the eyes, and the rest of the make-up is soft and pretty

KEYNOTES OF THE AUDREY HEPBURN LOOK

Dramatic full false lashes and lashings of mascara are a must for this wide-eyed look.

The eyebrows must have a sharply defined arch to frame the face.

Use powder eyeshadow in shades of gray and define the socket well to give the eyes depth.

The focus is on the eyes, so keep the pout pretty in soft pink, peach, or nude.

The skin needs a velvety, luminous finish.

The apples of the cheeks should be lightly flushed in natural peachy pink tones.

Top tip Ultrafine powder with light-reflecting particles sets the make-up and gives the skin a luminous glow. Blend it well with a large soft brush and circular motions for a polished velvety finish.

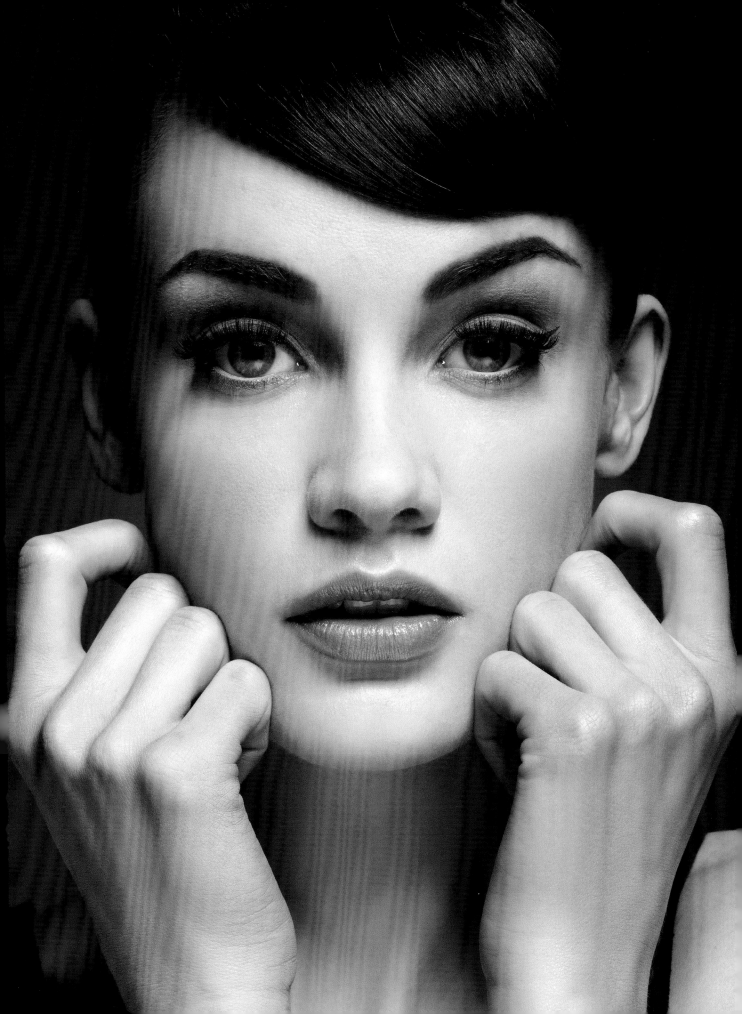

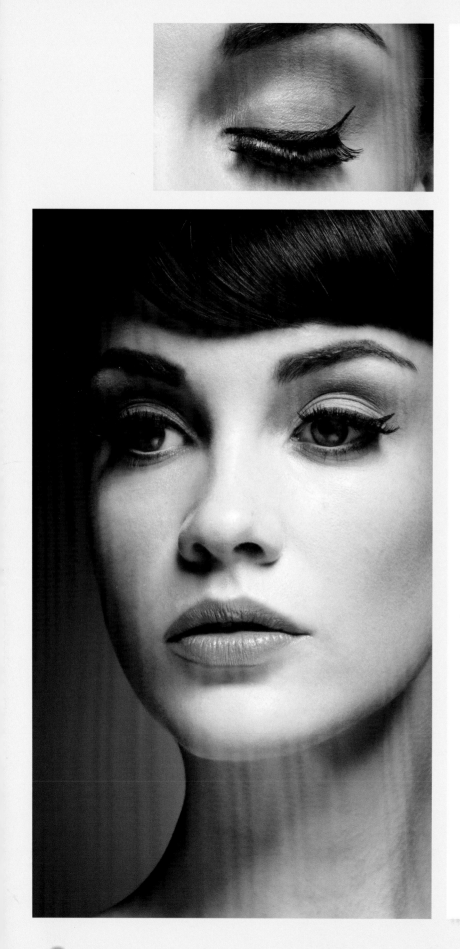

EYES Dramatic eyes with long full lashes

1 Fill the brows in with a matching brow pencil to create a full shape, and concentrate on accentuating the arch. Blend a little highlighter just beneath the hairs for extra definition.

2 Prime the eyelid to create a neutral base and use a nude pencil along the waterline to brighten and open up the eyes.

3 Apply a powder eyeshadow one shade lighter than your skin tone all over the lid.

4 Use a light gray eyeshadow to deepen the socket crease and then blend a little along the lower lash line at the outer corners.

5 Using a brown gel liner, draw along the upper lash line from the inner corner. Just before you reach the outer corner, draw a flick up toward the end of the brow.

6 Curl the lashes and coat them with black mascara. Apply full false lashes to accentuate the wide-eyed look.

SKIN Softly luminous skin

7 Use a mattifying primer to create a smooth shine-free base. Then even out the skin with a medium-coverage foundation and conceal any blemishes or undereye circles. Set the make-up with light-reflecting translucent powder.

8 Add subtle color to the face by brushing a soft, clear pink blush over the apples of the cheeks and blending it up toward the temples.

LIPS Light peachy pink lips

9 Exfoliate the lips and apply balm to create a smooth base.

10 Outline the lips with a soft pink lip liner, then color in the shape. Apply another coat of balm and blend it well with a lip brush.

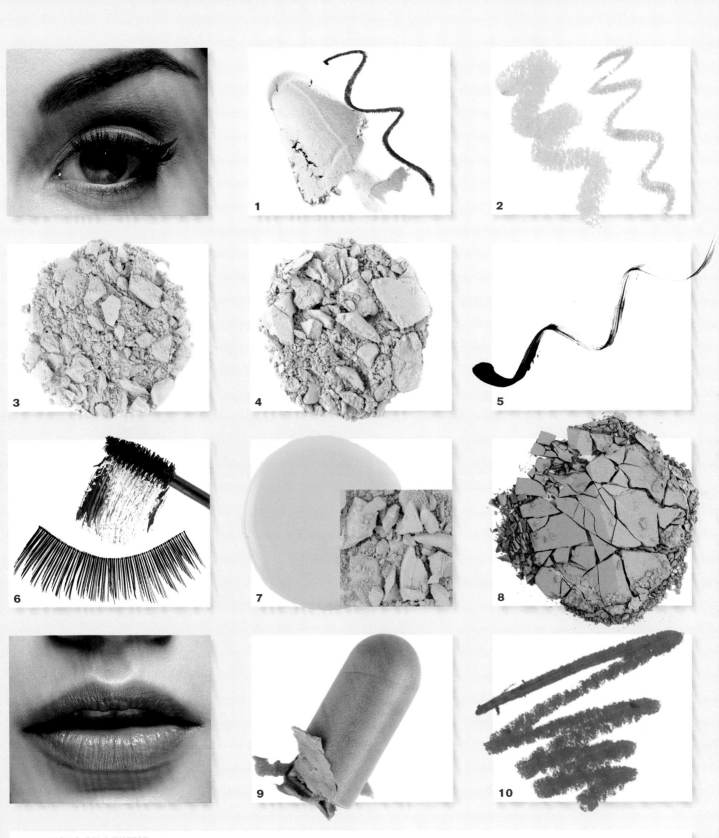

VARIATIONS ON A THEME

For a more natural and wearable version of this look, leave off the false lashes—just curl your lashes and coat them with mascara.

If your skin has yellow undertones, use taupe or light brown eyeshadow instead of gray, warm up your cheeks with apricot blush or bronzer, and use an apricot-toned nude lip color.

timeless look of

Ava Gardner

Considered one of the most beautiful women of her time, Ava Gardner began her movie career with a host of small roles before becoming one of Hollywood's brightest stars of the 1940s and 1950s. She had a classic heart-shape face with softly sculpted cheekbones, large eyes, and full lips that were invariably painted a sophisticated red. Framed by neatly arched brows, her eyes were subtly defined, with the outer third accentuated with shimmery eyeshadow and false lashes.

Ava Gardner's sultry beauty is easy to emulate with precisely painted red lips, polished skin and contoured cheekbones.

KEYNOTES OF THE AVA GARDNER LOOK

\# Full, glossy red lips are the epitome of Hollywood glamour. Draw the outline precisely but keep the shape natural and blend the gloss with a lip brush for a light all-over sheen.

\# Brows must arch softly with the highest point two-thirds of the way along, tapering gradually to a point at the outer corners.

\# Keep eyeliner thin and precise for subtle definition.

\# Accentuate the outer third of the eye to draw the focus upward and outward and make the eyes look farther apart.

\# Contour the cheeks, using matte bronzer to deepen the hollows and highlighter to bring the cheekbones forward.

Top tip To make your lips look fuller, after priming them, use a waxy red lip liner to draw just outside the natural outline, taking care to make the bow precise and the shape symmetrical. Fill in the color and blend with a lip brush. Then apply lipstick and top with red gloss.

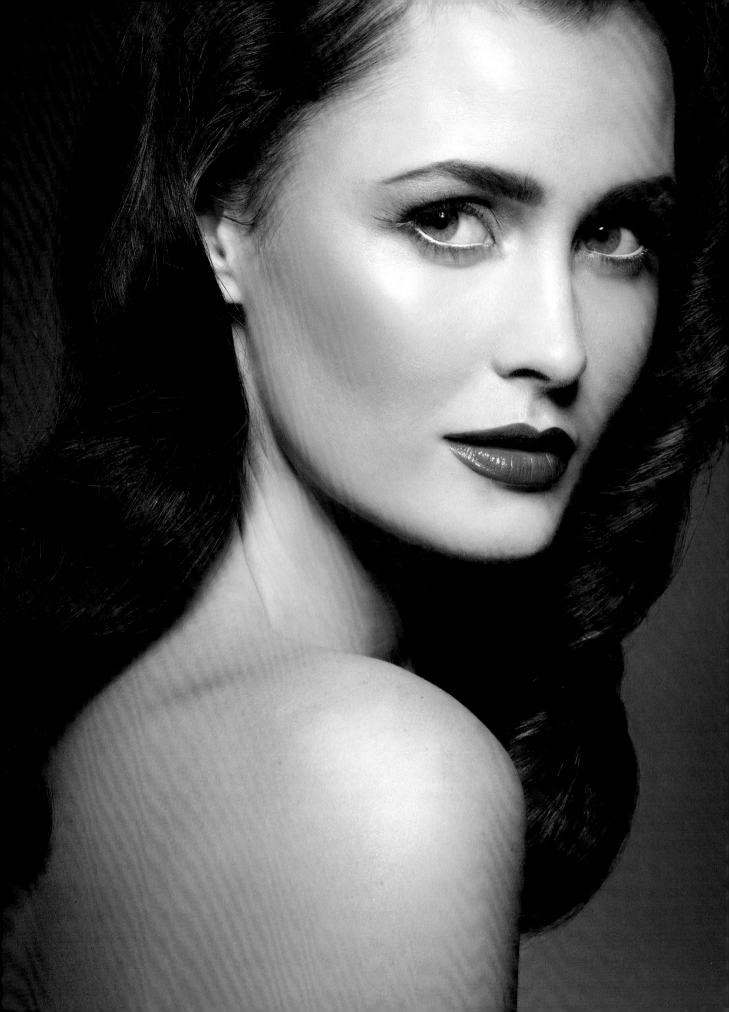

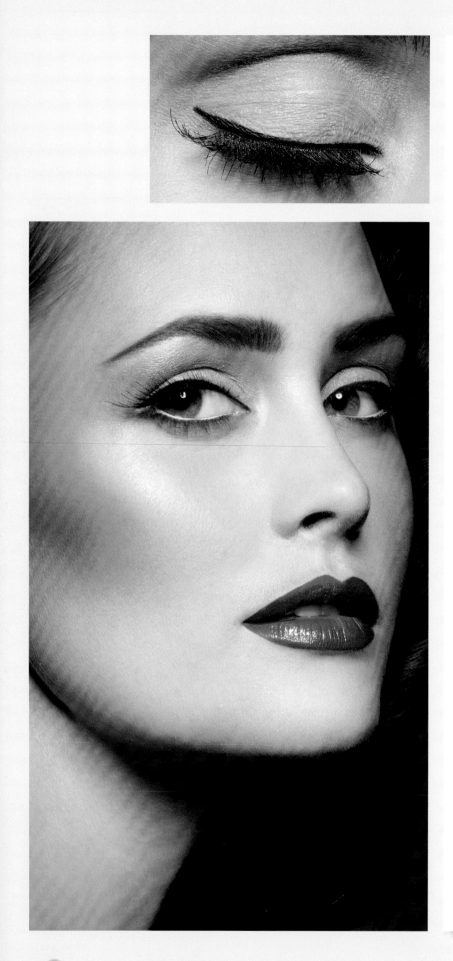

EYES Subtly defined wide-apart eyes

1 Use a natural brow powder to create a neat arch two-thirds of the way along the eye, tapering it to a point.

2 Prime the lid to create a smooth, neutral base. Use a white or nude eyeliner along the inner rim to brighten and open up the eyes.

3 Brush a nude powder eyeshadow over the lid and up to the browbone. Then define the socket with a soft pearl taupe eyeshadow. Blend it from the lashes at the outer third of the eye, up and out toward the bottom of the brow. Blend a little eyeshadow under the bottom lashes to create a shadow.

4 Draw a fine line of black pencil or gel eyeliner along the upper lash line, starting at the inner corner and taking it horizontally just beyond the end of the lashes at the outer corner.

5 Curl the lashes and coat them with mascara. Apply corner lashes to emphasize the outer part of the eyes.

SKIN Polished skin and sculpted cheeks

6 Use a primer to create a smooth base. Then blend medium-coverage foundation where you need it and cover any undereye circles or blemishes with concealer. Set with translucent powder, polishing it well with a large soft brush.

7 Contour the cheeks by blending matte bronzer just under the cheekbones and along the hairline.

8 Blend cream highlighter along the cheekbones, the bridge of the nose, and under the arches of the brows.

LIPS Full glossy Hollywood-red lips

9 Exfoliate the lips and then prime them with my Lip Perfector or foundation.

10 Outline the lips with a waxy lip liner that matches your lipstick. Fill in the shape and blend it with a lip brush.

11 Paint red lipstick over the top with the lip brush and then add a dab of red gloss and blend.

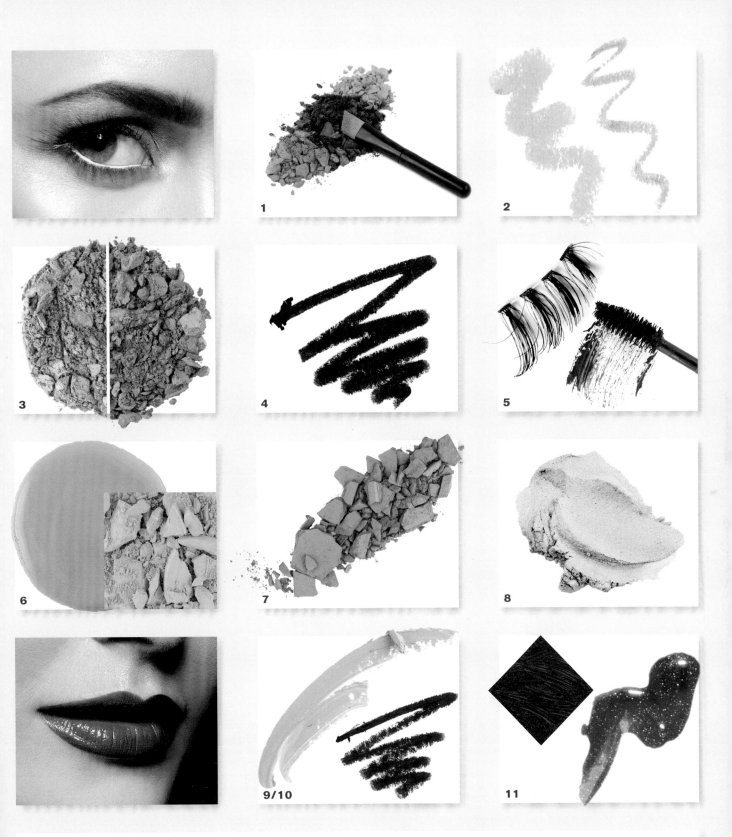

VARIATIONS ON A THEME

\# For enhanced lashes that look really natural, use individual lashes instead of corner lashes and apply just a few on the outer third of the eye for extra length and thickness.

\# Instead of pencil or gel eyeliner, you could use a darker toning eyeshadow, such as chocolate brown, along the lash line, blending it into the taupe eyeshadow on the rest of the lid. This would give a softer, smoky definition to the eyes.

timeless look of

Grace Kelly

A captivating beauty with natural poise, Grace Kelly made a seamless transition from Queen of the Silver Screen to Princess Grace of Monaco when she married Prince Rainier III in 1956. Her perfectly groomed look is perennially popular, chic, and very wearable. Her make-up was natural, with the emphasis usually being on bright lips in peach shades or bold red. Her eyes were kept simple, with a subtle wash of neutral eyeshadow, soft brown pencil liner for definition and neat but full brows. Underpinning the look was a flawless complexion with naturally flushed cheeks.

Grace Kelly's understated look is one of my favorites—serene and elegant, it's a timeless classic that is both youthful and sophisticated.

KEYNOTES OF THE GRACE KELLY LOOK

Concentrate on achieving a perfect base with natural-looking radiant skin.

This is no-make-up make-up with a pop of color on the lips, so keep the rest of the face as natural as possible with a subtle palette of neutral tones that blend well with the skin.

Eye make-up must be soft with no hard lines. Use brown pencil eyeliner instead of gel or liquid and blend it with a smudger.

Define the sockets with a darker toning eyeshadow, blending it well to create a shadow effect.

Make a focus of the lips with creamy moisturizing lipsticks in shades of peach or red.

Top tip If your natural lashes are sparse, use individual false lashes to add thickness and length in the least obvious way.

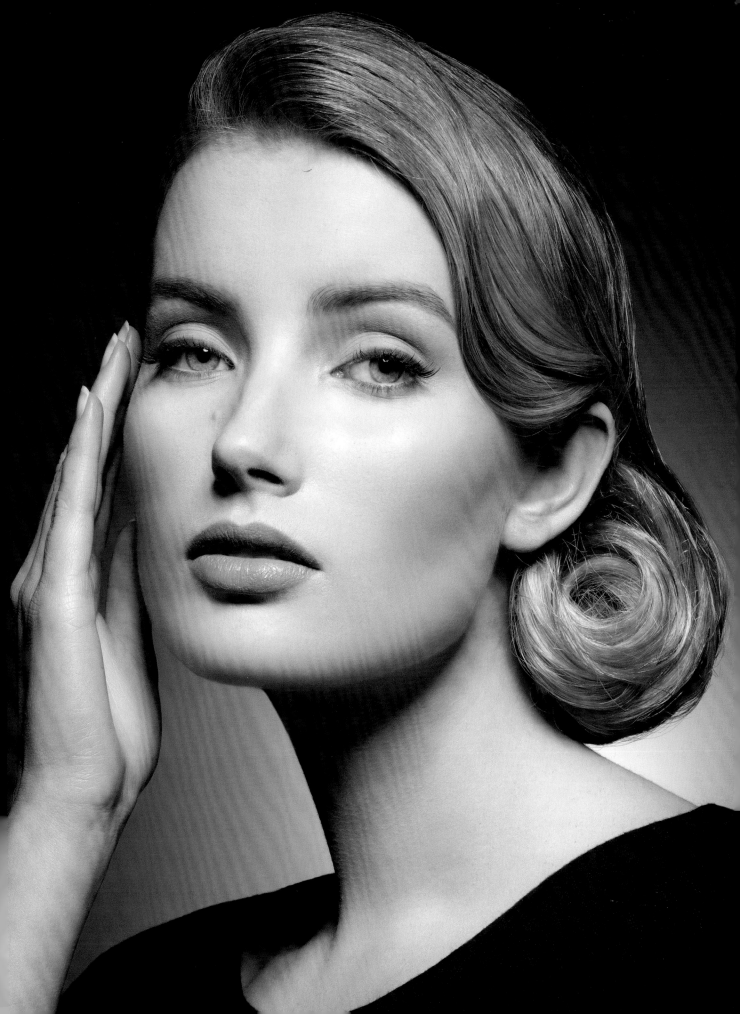

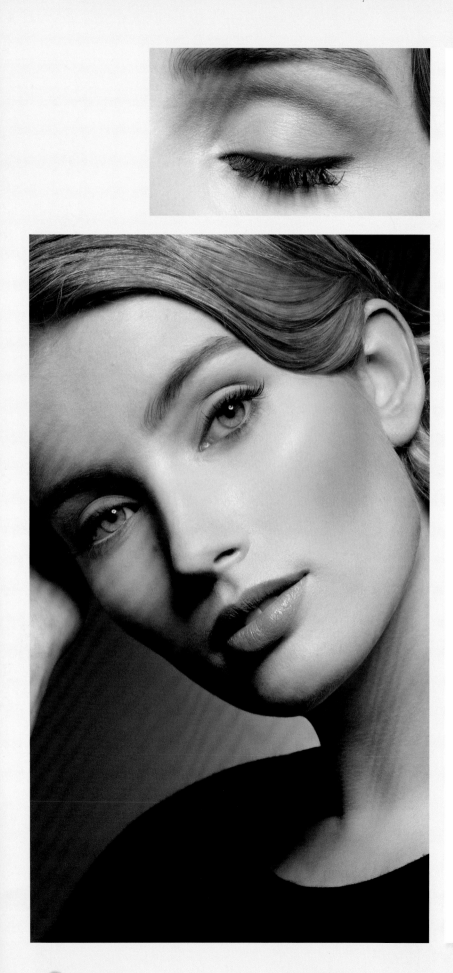

EYES Understated neutral eyes

1 Brush the brows into shape and fill in any gaps with matching brow powder to make them look naturally full.

2 Prime the eyelid to create a smooth base and conceal any redness. Use a nude eyeliner along the waterline to brighten and open up the eyes.

3 Use an eyeshadow one shade lighter than your skin tone all over your lid, up to the browbone.

4 Buff a taupe powder eyeshadow into the socket to give the eyes depth.

5 Using a brown pencil eyeliner, draw along the upper lash line from the inner corner and extend the line horizontally at the outer corner, taking it just beyond the end of the lashes.

6 Curl the lashes and coat them with black mascara.

SKIN Flawless and radiant complexion

7 Use a mattifying primer to create a smooth base and then even out your skin with a light-coverage radiance-boosting foundation. Use a creamy concealer under the eyes and on any blemishes, if you need to. Set with translucent powder, blending it well with a soft brush.

8 Softly contour the cheeks with a peachy nude powder blush.

9 Blend cream highlighter along the cheekbones and under the browbones.

LIPS Creamy peach lips

10 Exfoliate your lips and apply a waxy lip balm to create a smooth base.

11 Using a lip brush for a precise finish, apply creamy peach lipstick, working from the outside in.

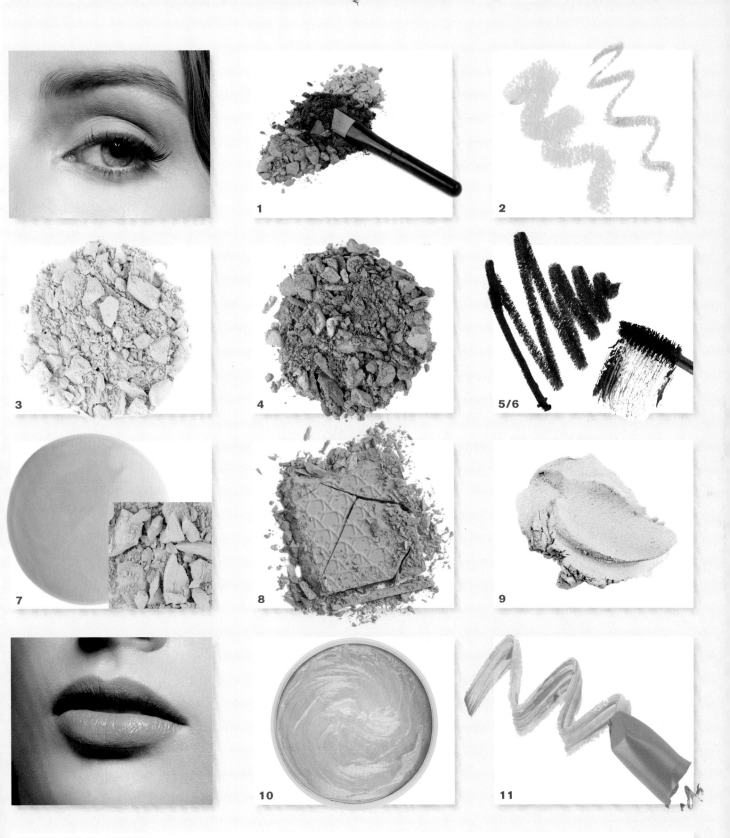

VARIATIONS ON A THEME

\#   For more drama, use red lipstick instead of peach—it's still a Grace Kelly classic. Choose a rich creamy texture with a light satin finish that will make your lips look really hydrated.

\#   If your skin is olive or deep, try a peach or apricot colorwash on your eyes, with a toning brown defining the sockets, and use bronzer to warm up your cheeks.

timeless look of
Sophia Loren

Sultry and sensuous, Italian actress Sophia Loren has been a beauty icon since she was a starlet in the 1950s. Her trademark cat-shaped eyes were achieved by applying liquid liner around the whole eye, meeting in a point at both corners. False lashes followed the eyeliner, extending beyond the lash line to accentuate the elongated shape. Eyeshadow, usually in soft brown, was blended over the lid and above the crease. Her strong brows were shaped into a rounded arch and brushed up for a textured finish. White pencil eyeliner along the waterline was another feature. Her cheekbones were sculpted in peach and her full lips were often lightly glossed in nude, pink, or soft brown.

Sophia Loren's sex-siren make-up is all about the dramatic eye shape, created with thick liquid liner that flicks up and out to give the illusion of elongated almond-shaped eyes.

KEYNOTES OF THE SOPHIA LOREN LOOK

The elongated cat's-eye shape was Sophia Loren's calling card. Use liquid or gel liner boldly to create the accentuated upward and outward flick.

For maximum drama, apply false lashes to extend beyond the lash line to really lengthen the eyes.

Use shades of brown eyeshadow to color the lids and deepen the socket crease. Choose warm browns if your skin has yellow undertones and cooler earthy browns if your skin has red undertones.

White eyeliner along the waterline brightens the eyes and makes them look larger. It also makes the black eyeliner look sharper.

For a full pout, keep lips soft and lightly glossy in shades of nude, soft pink, or brown.

Top tip Drawing the eye shape with pencil liner first not only means you can get the shape right and use that as a guide when applying the trickier gel or liquid liner, but it also intensifies the liner and gives it greater staying power.

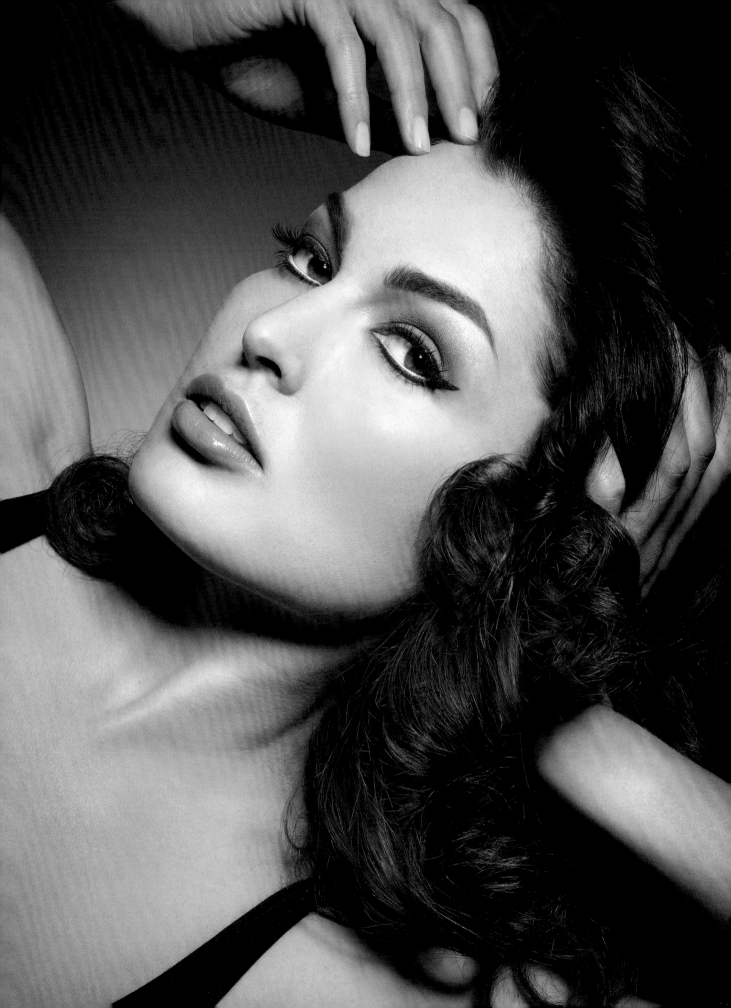

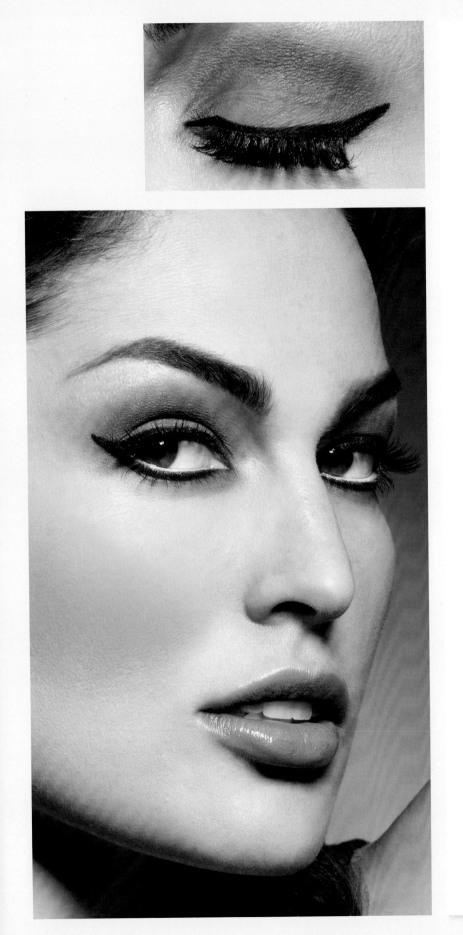

EYES The trademark cat's eye

1 Brush the brows up, then use an angled brow brush and natural powder to create texture as you fill in any gaps. Create a blunt end at the inner corner and an elegant arch tapering to a point at the outer corner.

2 Prime the eyelid to create a smooth and neutral base. Fill in the waterline with nude or white eyeliner.

3 Apply a warm brown eyeshadow from the upper lash line to the socket, then darken and define the crease.

4 Use a black pencil eyeliner to draw under the bottom lashes. Curve the line up and out at the outer corner, taking it toward the end of the brow. Draw along the upper lash line, starting at the inner corner and joining up with the bottom line. Fill in the triangle shape to create a flick in the outer corner. Go over the shape with black gel or liquid liner.

5 Apply lots of mascara to the top and bottom lashes and add a set of full false lashes for drama.

SKIN Glowing skin with contoured cheekbones

6 Apply a hydrating primer to create a smooth base, and even out the skin with a medium-coverage foundation. Use a creamy concealer to cover any blemishes or undereye shadows and then set with translucent powder.

7 Contour under the cheekbones and along the hairline with matte bronzer.

8 Brush a soft rose powder blush lightly over the cheekbones to create a natural flush.

9 Blend cream highlighter along the cheekbones, the bridge of the nose, and under the arches of the brows.

LIPS Natural full pout

10 Exfoliate the lips and moisturize with lip balm to create a smooth base. Then apply a sheer nude lipstick for a soft, healthy-looking finish.

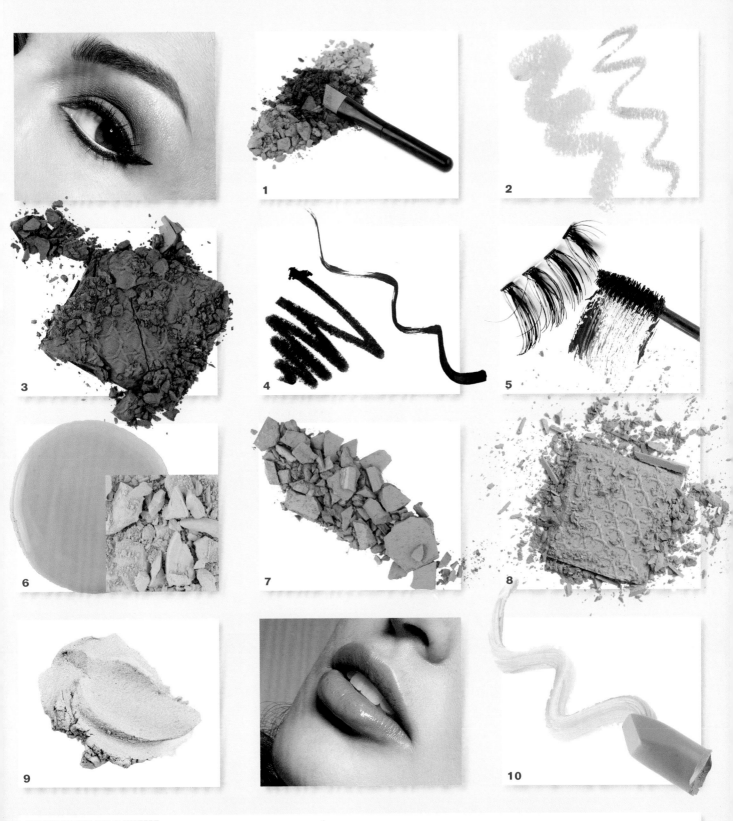

VARIATIONS ON A THEME

\# You can make the eye make-up as extreme as you wish. For a toned-down version, draw a finer outline of eyeliner, use lighter shades of eyeshadow and add individual false lashes rather than a full set.

\# Vamp it up with deeper lipstick and a touch of gloss.

2
PROBLEM SOLVER

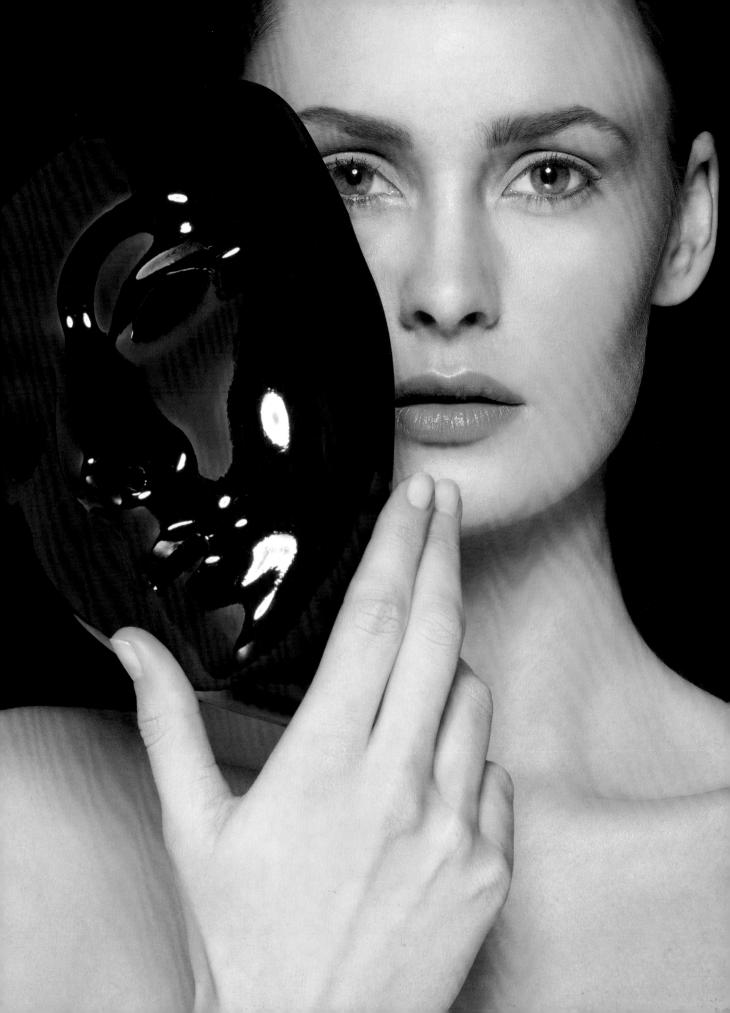

maintaining radiant skin

Naturally radiant skin is what every woman longs to have. If your skin is great, you automatically feel better about yourself and this confidence makes your inner beauty shine through.

The largest organ in the body, the skin is often the first place that signs of any imbalance in your lifestyle or diet manifest themselves. If your skin flares up, breaks out or is drier or oilier than usual, it is often a sign that something is out of kilter. Understanding your skin's behavior and how to address it is the first step to ensuring you have gorgeous skin every day. Although it's part of my role as a make-up artist to make skin look the best it can, I don't claim to be a skincare expert. So, to bring you the most up-to-date advice and information on the subject, I consulted my friend, beauty specialist and skincare technician Sarah Chapman, one of London's most sought-after facialists.

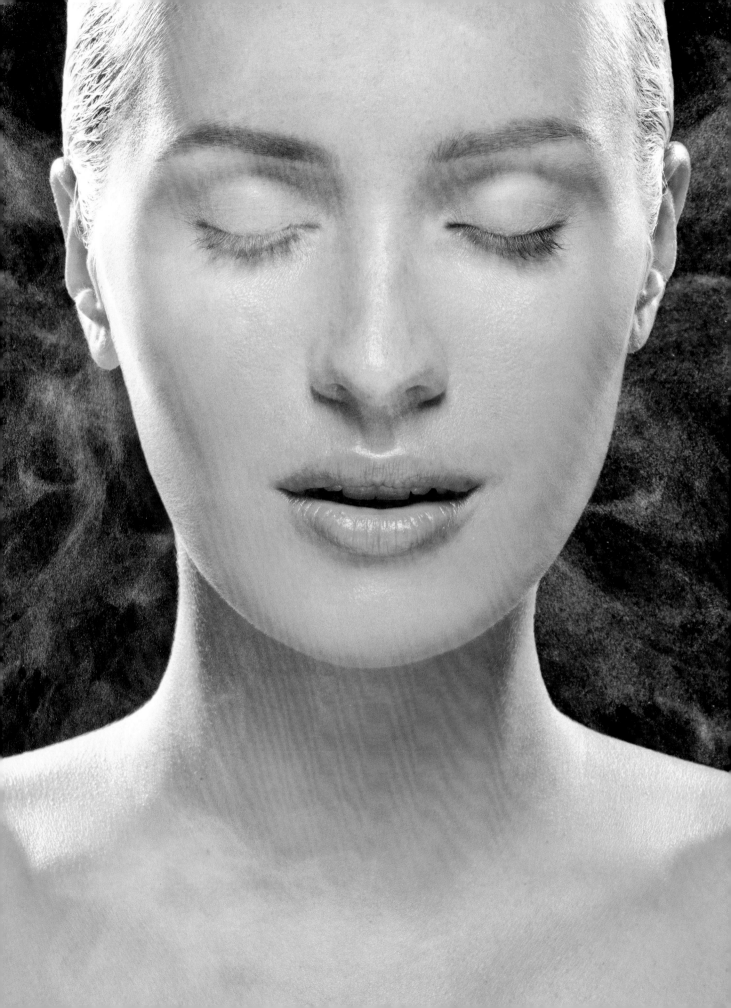

KEY PRINCIPLES FOR RADIANT SKIN

Cleanse well

So many people don't focus enough on cleansing. With today's long-wear make-up formulas, it is more important than ever to cleanse the skin thoroughly but without stripping it of its natural oils. In addition to the make-up we apply, dirt and grime from our polluted atmosphere attach themselves to the skin and make it dull and congested. Cleansing the skin thoroughly of surface dirt and dead cells keeps it healthy, as well as ensuring that it receives maximum benefits from any skincare products you use.

Take an Omega Oil supplement

Look for skincare products containing omega oils and take a supplement—you will see a massive improvement in your skin within three weeks. Found in flax seed and fish-oil supplements, omega oils are essential for cell health, as they strengthen cell membranes and help to keep cells intact, plump, and resilient. If your skin has been exposed to some kind of irritation, omega oils will help to rebuild and repair it.

Apply UV protection

UVA rays—the skin-damaging rays that cause cell destruction and aging—can penetrate glass and are harmful to the skin all year round, not just on sunny days. Rays from computer screens and fluorescent lighting may also assault the skin on a daily basis. Using a moisturizer with SPF every morning is a good starting point for protecting your skin, but when you are outside in the sun, regular reapplication of sun cream is essential. Using an inexpensive cream that you slather on regularly is preferable to eking out an expensive product.

Keep your skin hydrated

Skin that is dehydrated can look years older than it is, as the resulting fine lines make it look dull and accentuate wrinkles. Moisturizing well can transform the appearance of skin, making it look fresher, dewy, and plump, as it reflects the light more. Look for products containing Hyaluronic Acid, which is a real moisture magnet.

Look at your diet

Look after yourself from the inside out (see pages 162–7). One of the main things to avoid is sugar (especially the refined sugars found in cakes, candies, and cookies), which causes glycation in the skin, damaging collagen and accelerating the aging process. Caffeine is also bad for the skin. Like any artificial stimulant, it causes imbalance at a cellular level and is very dehydrating—you should drink at least two glasses of water for every cup of coffee. Alcohol is also dehydrating, as well as being full of sugar, and it breaks down energy-giving B vitamins, making you feel sluggish. Rehydrating with water and taking a Vitamin B supplement will help your body to metabolize a moderate intake of alcohol.

Use skincare products containing Vitamin A

Natural levels of Vitamin A in the skin reduce over time, and UV light and stress contribute to its breakdown. It is important to drip-feed a dose of Vitamin A into your skin every day, as it helps to strengthen cells and support the skin. Vitamin A is available in various forms— oil-based Retinyl Palmitate can pass easily through the lipid pathways of the skin without causing surface irritation; alcohol-based Retinol is very effective, but can be irritating to the skin's surface; while Retin-A, the dermatologist-prescribed acid form, has a peeling effect but delivers a high dose of Vitamin A, ideal for the complete rejuvenation of damaged skin. All forms of Vitamin A are converted into Retinoic Acid in the body, so whichever form you use, the effect will be similar at a cellular level.

top three skincare myths

1
People have "skin types." I believe in skin condition, which is affected by lifestyle, stress and seasonal and hormonal changes, and which can relatively easily be brought back into balance.

2
Natural products are gentle and anyone with sensitive skin should choose them over cosmeceuticals. In fact, natural extracts can be quite powerful and often cause more irritation than synthetically created ingredients. Cosmeceuticals are lab-controlled, but if something is derived from a plant, we have no idea how potent it is. In addition, many people are allergic to plant extracts or certain essential oils. Cosmeceuticals are not necessarily harsh and can deliver active ingredients in a controlled way to benefit the skin's health.

3
Oil-based products shouldn't be used on oily skin. Conversely, because oil has a natural affinity with oily skin, it can work with the skin, easily penetrating it and delivering its active ingredients. Oily skin will readily accept oil that is applied (think how oil mixes with oil but not with water) and then it won't produce so much natural oil. The most important product in this respect is cleansing oil or balm, which glides onto the skin and cleanses gently without stripping it.

KNOW YOUR SKIN

Don't focus on "skin type," focus on what your skin is like now and see what changes you need to make to balance it.

The condition of your skin can change with a change of season or because of your diet, hormones, stress levels, and lifestyle. Someone who had very dry skin as a teenager may find this is not the case as they grow older, while oily skin may balance itself naturally.

how to self-diagnose your skin

After cleansing, leave your skin bare for a couple of hours.

Sensitive skin Skin sensitivity is an increasing concern, as lifestyle and stress can be contributing factors. However, many people think they have sensitive skin when they don't. If your skin responds with heat and redness when you apply a product, if you flush easily, or if touching your face leaves red marks that take a long time to go, you could have an underlying skin sensitivity.

Normal skin If your skin has a light sheen, you have good oil production.

Dry skin If your skin feels really tight and you are desperate to apply moisturizer, it is likely your skin is in a dry state.

Oily skin If your skin is really shiny, you could be producing too much oil. Press a tissue against the skin and see how much oil is absorbed.

Problem skin There is a big difference between having a few spots and suffering from acne, which can be painful and distressing. There are three grades of acne, from mild, where the skin has little pimples, to full-grade, where hard cysts are surrounded by inflamed skin that has a purple tone. Mild acne can be treated at home, but if you have full-grade acne, consult your doctor.

Dehydrated skin Take a looking glass to the window and hold it so that light falls crosswise onto your face. If your skin is dehydrated, you will see a crisscross of fine lines that make the surface seem scaly and dull. If your skin is hydrated, it will reflect the light and look smooth. Another easy test is to pinch the back of your hand and see how quickly the skin bounces back. If you are adequately hydrated, the skin is as elastic as it can be and should bounce back immediately.

T-zone The area across the forehead and down the nose and chin is oilier than the cheeks and often prone to shine, blocked pores, and blackheads (see page 178).

Eyelids The thin skin around the eyes and on the eyelids is prone to sensitivity and redness, which can be aging and make you look tired.

Around the nose The skin on either side of the nose often shows signs of broken capillaries and thread veins, which cause redness.

Cheeks The fragile skin on the cheeks is drier than the rest of the face, and flaky patches can appear. Redness is also a common problem.

Chin As well as being greasy and prone to spots, the chin often suffers from redness.

how to balance your skin

Dry skin

A lack of oils, as opposed to moisture (see Dehydrated skin, below), makes dry skin feel tight. It needs more oil, preferably both internally and externally. Dry skin responds really well to massaging oil into the skin and benefits from a good lipid-rich barrier cream. Gentle oil-based cleansing will ensure that you don't strip the skin of the little natural oil it has.

Oily or breakout-prone skin

The key thing is not to overcleanse. Don't use products that are stripping, such as foaming cleansers or alcohol-based products, because your skin will then produce more oil to counteract this. Use an oil-based cleanser and, if you like your skin to have a squeaky-clean feel, wash it off with a light wash or milk. If you are prone to spots, breakouts, or blackheads, look for products containing Salicylic Acid, which helps to de-clog the pores, lifting out the plugs of sebum and bacteria. Don't forget to moisturize oily skin—you may have a lot of oil, which creates sheen, but a lack of hydration shows up as a crisscross, scaly surface.

Dehydrated skin

Initially, focus on gentle exfoliation to get rid of the layer of dead cells on the surface. Use products with an ingredient like Hyaluronic Acid, which locks moisture into the skin. Dehydrated skin requires a two-pronged internal and external approach, and essential fats are needed to ensure the body retains water. If you drink 8 glasses (2 litres) of water a day and moisturize well but still have dehydrated skin, look at your fat intake—your good omegas. Support dehydrated skin with antibacterial ingredients, as the barrier of protection will be compromised and, if the skin is broken, bacteria may penetrate, causing itching, redness, scaliness, or pimples.

Sensitive skin

Treat the skin gently and focus on rebuilding and defending it. Look for ingredients like Beta Glucan and stem cells, and take an omega oil supplement and probiotics, which are very restoring. Avoid AHAs (Alpha Hydroxy Acids), exfoliants, and heavy or synthetic perfumes, which can trigger a reaction. Increase hydration levels to reduce inflammation. Make sure the skin is always protected and don't overlook the little things. For example, when you take a bath, prevent trans-epidermal water loss by applying a hydrating mask; if you have had a treatment like a peel, don't lean over a boiling kettle or an open oven door and subject your face to a sudden whoosh of hot air, as this can break the capillaries and exacerbate sensitivity.

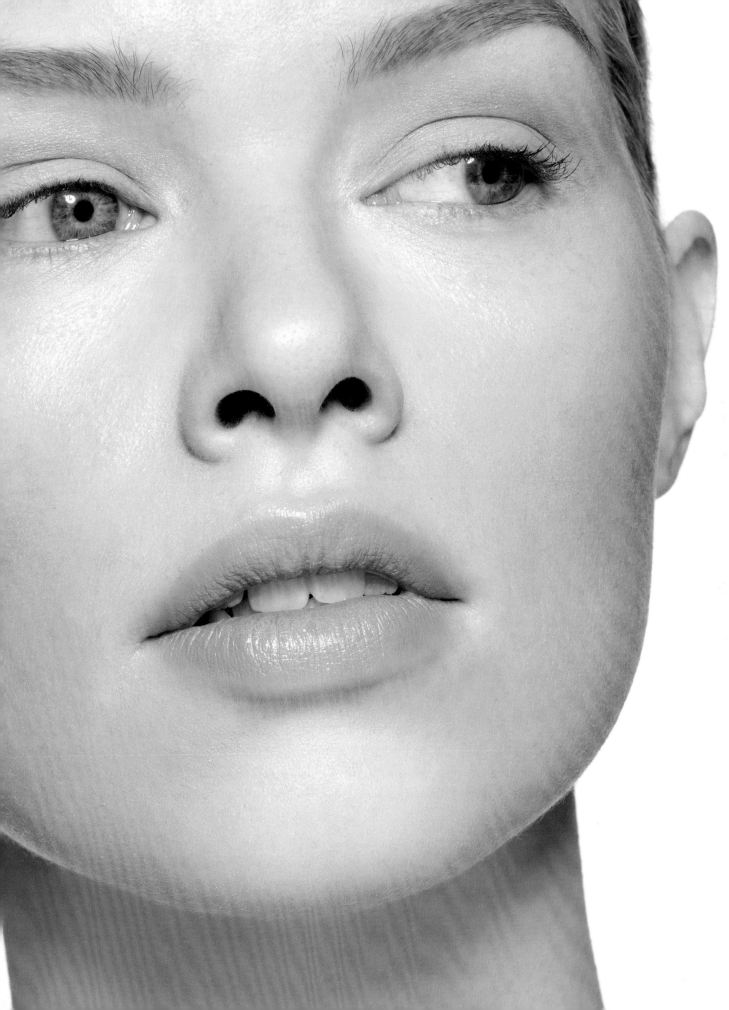

HOW TO KEEP SKIN LOOKING **DEWY**

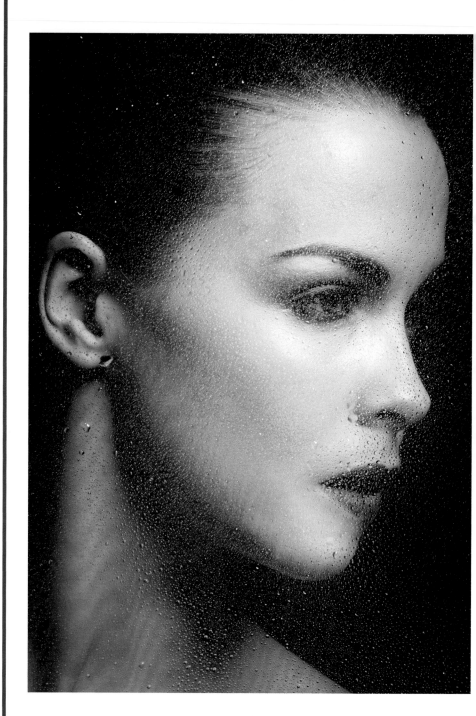

Dewy skin has a fresh, youthful bloom that makes it look radiant, plump, and healthy. It feels soft and is smoother and less lined than dehydrated skin, which can look drawn and dull.

On average the body loses around 16 ounces (600ml) of water a day by evaporation through the skin. If the water that has been lost is not replaced, the underlying tissue, known as the dermis layer, cannot transfer as much moisture to the outer layer, the epidermis, which results in dry and sometimes flaky skin. Over time, dehydration causes the skin to lose its elasticity and radiance. It brings about premature aging by encouraging wrinkles and superficial lines to form, especially around the eye area. Picture a grape shriveling up to a raisin.

Some causes of dehydration

Poor cleansing Cleansers or soap that leave skin "squeaky clean" or feeling tight are dehydrating, especially soap, as it is alkaline which is harsh to the skin.

Sun damage Continual sun exposure breaks down the skin's dermal tissues, which affect the transfer of moisture to the epidermis.

Temperature extremes Exposure to cold wind, air conditioning, and central heating can all deprive the skin of vital moisture. This slows down the renewal process—the shedding of dead skin cells to make way for fresh new skin—often leaving a dry, taut, flaky surface.

Scrubs An overuse of scrubs, or using harsh scrubs, can break down cell cohesion in certain skin types; this reduces the skin's ability to retain moisture and places the capillaries at risk.

Hot showers Hot water and friction remove sebum, the skin's natural oil, from the surface of the skin, causing capillary damage and dehydration. Always wash your face using lukewarm water.

Medication Cold and flu remedies that dry up mucus also dehydrate the skin's surface.

Poor diet An excessive intake of salt and drinks that are high in caffeine and sugar.

Neglect Failure to drink enough fluids and not applying protective creams regularly.

HELPFUL HINTS

\# Cleanse with a gentle oil-based product and wipe it off with a muslin cloth soaked in warm water. The cloth will gently exfoliate, while the heat will open the pores, allowing moisturizer to sink deeper into the skin.

\# Facial oil hydrates the skin to a deeper level than a cream or lotion. Its natural ingredients penetrate the skin's layers, delivering moisture, vitamins, and essential fatty acids. Facial oil can restore dry, chapped, and itchy skin, but is most successful in keeping the skin elastic and youthful-looking when applied regularly.

:) GOOD DRINKS

Water—drink at least eight glasses or 8 glasses (2 litres) of still water a day

Herbal teas—they contain beneficial antioxidants

Hot water with lemon—extremely cleansing and a source of Vitamin C

:(BAD DRINKS

Anything with a high caffeine content

Sugary and fizzy drinks

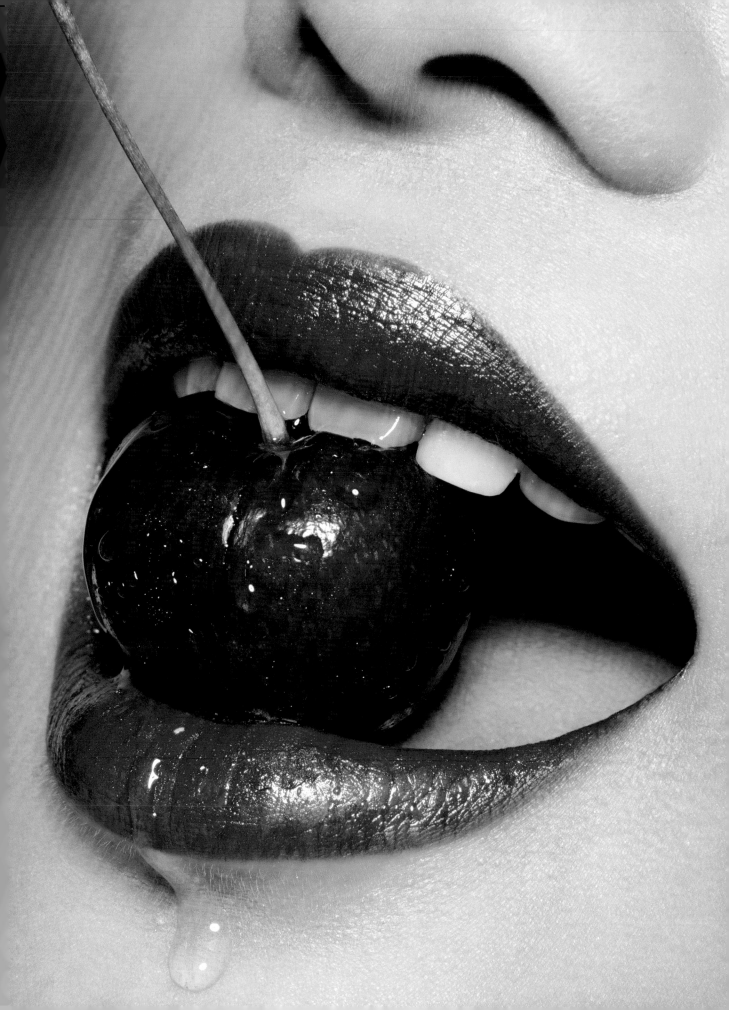

HEALTHY SKIN FROM THE INSIDE OUT

I have been to see many nutritionists because of problems with my digestion, but it wasn't until I saw the wonderful Petronella Ravenshear that my condition was solved. She changed everything and turned my life around, which is why I am sharing her knowledge with you here.

The buzzwords for gorgeous skin: hydrate, nourish, detoxify, sleep, repair

your second skin

The gut lining is a very thin skin, just one layer thick. Like the skin on the face, it acts as a barrier, allowing some things in and other things out. Like a mirror, our outer skin reflects the state of this inner skin—if it is functioning properly, our skin will be balanced and healthy—which is why we talk about beauty coming from the inside.

When the gut lining is intact, it prevents toxins from entering the circulation while letting the nutrients in—think of very sophisticated sliding doors. If the gut lining is damaged, it becomes leaky, meaning that partly digested food proteins escape into the bloodstream. This can trigger food intolerances, as the immune system thinks the proteins are enemies and creates antibodies to attack them.

:) GOOD FOR THE GUT LINING

High-strength, nondairy probiotic bacteria—this is the single most important thing to maintain the integrity of the gut

:(DAMAGING TO THE GUT LINING

Antibiotics

Emotional stress

Too much alcohol

Infections

GOLDEN RULE

Good nutrition and beautiful skin go hand in hand. If we give our bodies the right amount of water and the right nutrition, we enable it to function to the best of its ability, cleansing our system of waste products and processing the nutrients required at a cellular level. Everything you eat and drink that is good for your skin and makes you beautiful is equally good for your health, and vice versa.

what to eat

Everything that we put into our body has either an inflammatory effect or an anti-inflammatory effect. It's a question of getting the balance right. Too much inflammatory or acid-forming food can result in skin conditions such as eczema, psoriasis, dermatitis, acne, and rosacea. The simplest way to assess what you are eating and the effect it is likely to have on your skin and how you look is to ask yourself, "Is this a natural food?"

Think like a hunter-gatherer

Early man's diet consisted of vegetables, fruit, nuts, eggs, fresh meat, fish, and shellfish. There was no way to process grains or legumes to make them edible, there was no sugar, other than in fruits and honey, and no milk after weaning. The idea that we need to drink another animal's milk to get the calcium we need is absurd. Think of a cow with its enormous bones and what it eats—grass. Green vegetables are our most important source of calcium and magnesium. Most of us actually have too much calcium in our diets and not enough magnesium. Without magnesium, calcium is not taken into the bones but dumped in the soft tissue, where it builds up and causes problems (calcification), like limescale in a kettle.

If you have dry or oily skin

The most important thing for both dry and oily skin is, paradoxically, more oil—namely the essential omega 3 and omega 6 oils, which help to rebalance the skin and reduce inflammation. The modern diet is rich in omega 6 (which comes from plant oils, such as sunflower and rapeseed), but unless there is also enough omega 3 in our diet, these omega 6 oils make pro-inflammatory compounds and do not turn into the vitally important GLA (Gamma-linolenic acid).

COMMON COMPLAINTS THAT RESULT FROM A POOR DIET

Acne is often connected with polycystic ovarian syndrome (PCOS) and can be made worse by sugar. Make sure you are getting enough Omega 3 fats, which reduce inflammation. Stress affects hormone levels, so use de-stressing techniques such as meditation, yoga, and breathing exercises. Deficiencies in Zinc and Vitamin A can also be causes of acne.

Eczema is often the result of an allergy to milk, and may be helped both by avoiding dairy products and by taking probiotics.

Excessive hair on the face or body often goes hand in hand with acne and PCOS. Avoid sugar and beware of hidden sugars— for example, in products made with white flour, which contains very little fiber and so breaks down quickly into sugar in the bloodstream. Fruit is also high in sugar, so don't eat too much—stick to a handful of blueberries and an apple a day.

Psoriasis can be a sign that the liver is struggling with detoxification. There may be an overgrowth of yeast, such as candida, in the body, or problems with gluten digestion.

A puffy face and bloated stomach often go together. Bloating is frequently associated with allergies, mainly to dairy and gluten. The best remedy is to take probiotic bacteria and get your digestion functioning correctly.

Rosacea may be due to poor digestive chemistry, when not enough gastric acid is produced.

Superfoods and supplements

Antioxidant supplement
It is hard to get all we need through diet alone

Apples
Rich in antioxidants and pectin, a gut-friendly toxin-removing fiber

Blueberries
Rich in antioxidants

Broccoli
Another source of antioxidants and possibly the king of the superfoods: excellent for hormone balance and liver detoxification

Glucosamine
A beneficial supplement for healthy joints and skin

Magnesium
Used to make ATP, the energy currency of the cell, magnesium is essential to maintain energy levels—we need 500–1000mg a day, but a good diet contains only 150–200mg

Omega 3, 6, and 9 essential fatty acids
An anti-inflammatory that will help to improve skin, hair, nails, general health, energy levels, and concentration. Take a good-quality supplement and make sure it contains DHA as well as EPA (the two components of omega 3 fish oil), as the former is important for the skin. Udo's Choice Oil is an organic blend of unrefined nutritional oils that I particularly recommend

Sauerkraut and miso
Examples of healthy fermented foods

Vitamin C
It is hard to get sufficient from food alone. Choose a supplement with bioflavanoids, such as pomegranate, plum, and blueberry extracts

Vitamin D
An important supplement in areas where there is little sun, as sunlight stimulates the production of Vitamin D, needed to make cholesterol and to maintain a healthy immune system, bones, joints, and state of mind

Water
The number-one skin-friendly nutrient

PROBIOTIC BACTERIA

Probiotics are essential for a healthy digestive system. They make B vitamins, are anti-inflammatory, and they line the gut, helping to keep it intact and protect the immune system—80 percent of which is in the gut. Together with water and fiber, probiotic bacteria also keep the bowel working efficiently. They provide energy for peristalsis, which keeps bowel movements regular—if the bowels aren't emptied, toxins can be reabsorbed by the body and go back into circulation. (For this reason, colonics can be beneficial, especially for anyone prone to constipation.) Three-quarters of a stool is dead probiotic bacteria, which, along with the fiber in our diet, provide the bulk that is needed for a perfect stool. This is why we need to keep replacing them.

WHAT TO AVOID

Anything that is not meat, fish, chicken, eggs, nuts, seeds, fruit, or vegetables—it's as easy as that.

Blackened and processed meat, especially barbecued meat, which contains cancer-promoting compounds.

Chips and fries, although potatoes are fine now and then.

Citrus fruits can be quite allergenic and bananas are high in sugar, so keep these to a minimum; focus on berries, especially blueberries, and apples.

Dairy products, especially milk and cheese, which are hard to digest. If you must have milk, try coconut milk or almond milk—you can make your own by putting almonds in a blender with mineral water and then straining it.

Gluten-containing grains, such as wheat, rye, and barley, which are very hard to digest and can cause bloating.

Soya products, other than miso. Soy is allergenic, and unfermented soy interferes with thyroid function, which can result in weight gain, depression, dry skin, and constipation.

Sugar—the number one thing to avoid. An anti-nutrient, sugar actually uses up stores of vitamins and minerals when it is broken down and absorbed. It also speeds up glycation, which is when the collagen (a protein) in the skin stiffens, resulting in wrinkles and dehydration.

how to eat

Eat as regularly as possible, leaving at least five hours between meals. Combine different colors of fruit and vegetables—yellow and orange from carrots, squash, and peppers; green from all the green vegetables; purple from berries, cherries, purple sprouting broccoli, red cabbage, and eggplant. You can eat a mix of vegetables, but try not to mix different proteins in the same meal, and only have one type of fruit afterward. A mixture of proteins or fruits is harder for the body to digest.

HOW TO IMPROVE DIGESTION

It all comes down to the gut. If your digestion isn't working properly, you can't absorb the nutrients your body needs.

Eat slowly
Chew thoroughly
Eat fewer carbohydrates
Eat raw foods, which contain live enzymes
Exercise before eating

Petronella Ravenshear's mini menus

BREAKFAST

There is no reason to eat cereal or toast for breakfast. For increased energy levels and more calorie-burning, base your breakfast on protein. Good breakfasts include:

2 eggs, boiled, poached, or made into an omelette with green vegetables, such as spinach or broccoli, followed by an apple

Smoked salmon with green vegetables, such as a small avocado

Full-fat Greek yogurt with blueberries and flaked almonds or ground seeds

A handful of walnuts or almonds with an apple or some berries

Almond butter or tahini with carrot or celery sticks

Gluten-free oats (1oz/30g), soaked overnight in coconut milk, with a grated apple, a pinch of cinnamon, and a sprinkling of ground almonds

These are the supplements I use the most and get the best results with:

Symprove liquid and live probiotics

Bionutri all their products are excellent, especially their digestive enzyme Ecogest, their probiotic capsules Ecodophilus (more convenient than Symprove when you are traveling), and CT Plex, which is fabulous not only for skin but also for joints. Bionutri Vitamin C Complex comes with pomegranate and blueberry for maximum absorption

Allergy Research for their collagen powder Arthred, which is great for skin and joints

LUNCH

To keep you going for longer and with better energy levels, avoid carbohydrates (bread, pasta, rice, or potato). Instead combine protein (either meat, fish, eggs, shellfish, or chicken, but not a mixture) with salad and/or green vegetables. If you are in a hurry, buy prepared salads and sliced cooked chicken or turkey. Avocados are very nutritious and mushrooms are good for the immune system and, therefore, the skin.

DINNER

Combine vegetables with protein. Be adventurous with vegetables—make quick and easy stir-fries of different-colored vegetables (all contain different nutrients). Add lots of herbs, including chili and garlic if you like them, and either fish or chicken. Use coconut oil or olive oil for cooking.

Juicing makes you feel and look good

Vegetable juices give your body a powerful shot of pure minerals, vitamins, and nutrients that no other food or drink can provide. They are health in a glass and make me feel alive.

The way I see it, juicing simply makes sense—it's fresh and it's raw, so it must be full of live enzymes, vitamins, and minerals, which are undeniably good for us. Humans are the only animals that eat cooked food (apart from dogs and cats—and look who feeds them). Cooking destroys the nutrients that raw foods are packed full of, so even when you eat healthily, you are giving your body fuel but not flooding it with goodness.

I prefer green juices for their high chlorophyll and fiber content. Green vegetables are the most nutritionally dense and are high in antioxidants. Whatever you juice, make sure it's organic, and beware of adding fruit and vegetables with a high sugar content, such as carrots. Don't substitute juices for eating whole fruits and vegetables, either, as the fiber they contain is very important for overall health and feed the good bacteria in your gut.

Drinking a green juice every day gives you:

More energy

Clearer skin

Improved digestion and regular bowel movements

A body that is being nourished, not malnourished

I can't see myself ever going back to the days before juicing—it has changed my life for the better and now my whole family does it.

LITTLE DOS AND DON'TS FOR BEAUTY FROM THE INSIDE OUT

Do

Drink at least 8 glasses of still water a day
(think plum not prune)
Get enough sleep (repair and relaxation)
Ditch the sugar (who wants fat and wrinkly?)
Take digestive enzymes and probiotics
(beauty begins in the gut)
Eat an apple a day (and some blueberries)
Get daily exercise (walk everywhere you can)
Keep a food diary to keep track of your nutrition

Don't

Eat before you exercise
Drink too much water while you are eating
Snack between meals—rest your digestion
Drink too much alcohol—a glass of wine
a day is fine
Eat wheat (or any grains, as far as possible)
Focus on calories or a low-fat diet
Beat yourself up if you break the rules,
just start again!

FACT OR FICTION

Every month, it seems, new products and ingredients flood the market, supported with convincing write-ups that have women lining up at cosmetics counters and joining waiting lists for the next beauty-industry wonder. This can be costly as well as confusing, so I asked the advice of Sarah Chapman, my skincare guru.

the inside scoop on skincare

There are lots of ingredients that work at certain levels, but a product's efficacy depends on the concentration the manufacturers are using—and it is very hard to know that. Generally, the higher up an ingredient is on the ingredients list, the more of it the product contains—anything listed below fragrance will have a very minimal concentration. However, some ingredients are very powerful and are only needed in very small doses to be effective.

In fact, some become ineffective in larger doses, so the key to a product working well is for the manufacturers to find the correct levels for those compounds. In addition, some ingredients make others work better, so the synergy and fusion between ingredients is also an important factor. For example, Vitamin E recycles Vitamin C, so it lasts longer and has a better effect.

SKINCARE INGREDIENTS THAT REALLY WORK

Hyaluronic Acid, which helps the skin retain water, plumping and supporting it

Peptides, such as Matrixyl, Dermaxyl and Syn-ake, which stimulate the production of collagen

Stem-cell ingredients—the new buzzwords in the beauty industry, stem cells extracted from sea algae, plants, and flowers stimulate the production of collagen and help repair and strengthen the skin. New technology is looking at ways to extract the real life force of the plant—especially of algae or mountain flowers that grow in harsh conditions—and incorporate the purified form of the stem cells that keep the plants alive into skincare

Vitamins, especially A, C, and E. Vitamin A is the only skincare ingredient that the FDA (Food and Drug Administration) recognizes as truly anti-aging, as it has been proven to repair cells from UV damage and is prescribed by dermatologists to treat acne and other serious skin conditions

Antioxidants—Alpha Lipoic Acid, Co-Enzyme Q10, Carnosine, and Vitamins A, C, and E—which mop up damaging free radicals and optimize cell health

Sunscreen, which protects the skin against aging UVA rays as well as burning UVB rays

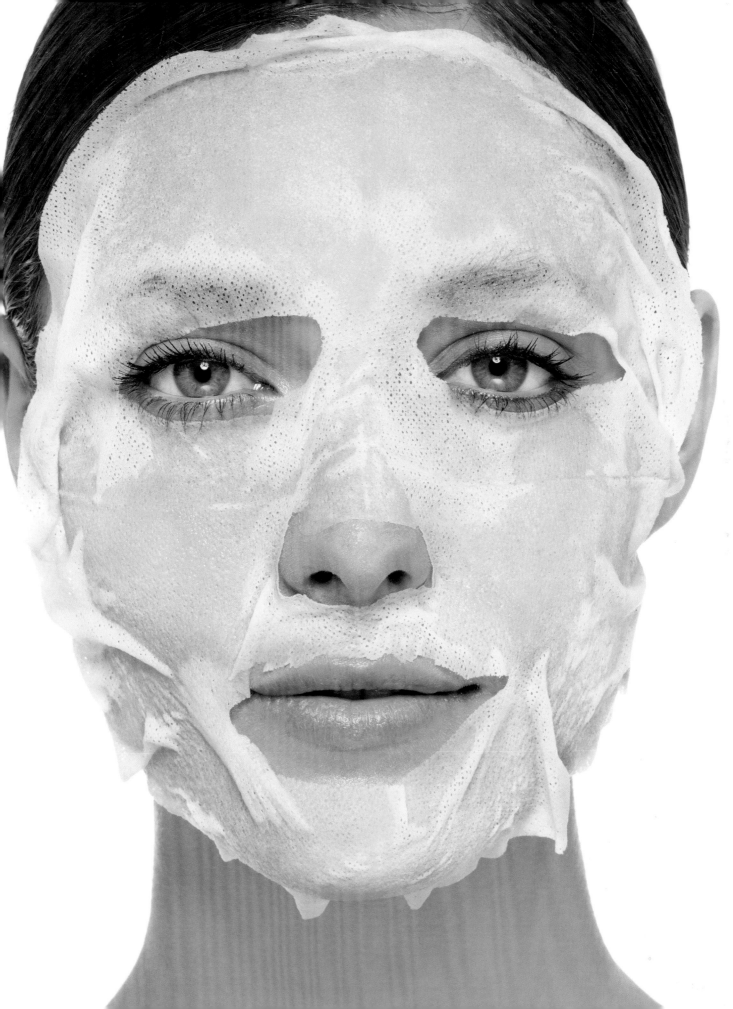

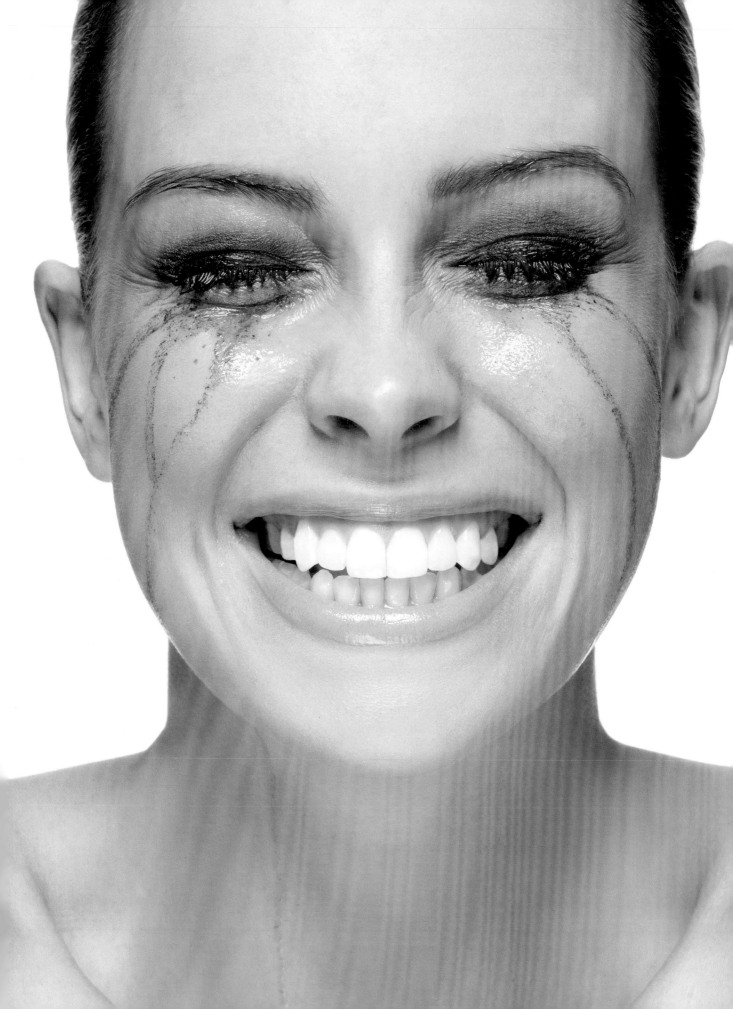

Sarah Chapman's advice on popular products

Cleansers In my skincare clinic we focus on oil-cleansing, a method that dates back years in Japan and is equally effective on dry, mature, and oily skins, as it helps to regulate natural sebum secretions. Soft oil-based balm is gentle enough to use on sensitive areas, even around the eyes, and melts away even the most stubborn long-lasting mascara when it is massaged in gently with little circular movements. When the skin is rinsed with warm water and gently patted dry, it will feel supple and refreshed.

Exfoliators Choose a very gentle exfoliator—no harsh, scratchy granules—and use it once or twice a week, depending on your skin. Always be gentle with your skin, never scrub or rub it.

Toners Some people love toners, but for me they are no more than a cooling freshener to sweep on the skin, although they can help to balance its pH. If you cleanse properly, you shouldn't need a toner to remove any residue, but if you want to use one, opt for an exfoliating or hydrating toner that offers an additional benefit.

Night treatment At night, the main concern for your skin is cellular response and renewal, whereas during the day it is defense. After cleansing at night, I recommend using an oil-type product, as you need something that penetrates and delivers all the active ingredients and goodies to your skin.

Eye creams Some people find eye cream too heavy, while others find gel too sticky and not nourishing enough, so opt for a texture somewhere in between, such as a serum. Eye creams are designed to treat the eye area differently from the rest of the face because the skin is very thin and delicate, with fewer oil glands. Using a product that is too rich and heavy can cause puffiness. The lids and underneath the eyes are subjected to a lot of facial expression and movement, so immobilizing peptides are worthwhile ingredients in eye creams.

Masks Use a mask whenever your skin needs an instant pick-me-up or an extra shot of hydration. If your skin is stressed, use an anti-inflammatory or clarifying mask.

Lip balms Look for a petroleum-free product. Petroleum-based lip balms form a protective film over your lips but don't moisturize them, so ultimately they make your lips drier and you have to keep reapplying. This is why Carmex and Vaseline become addictive. Shea butter is lovely for conditioning, softening, and nourishing the lips.

Daily moisturizer This is an essential product that you should use every morning to help lock moisture in the skin and form a seal of protection. Think of moisturizer like a coat—defending you against all the nasties in the environment, while also helping to keep everything underneath comforted.

★ **Top tip** There's an element of truth to "you get what you pay for," because the cost of the high-performing active ingredients pushes the retail prices up, but there is a limit to what can go into a product, so it is doubtful that a $500 serum is justifiable. At the higher end of the $5–$40 range, it is probably true to say that you will get a more sophisticated formula that will deliver better results.

SKINCARE REGIME

Instead of the traditional steps of cleanse, tone, moisturize, try: cleanse, serum, moisturize.

Sophisticated modern formulas mean that a cleanser should do the job without the need for a separate toner. Instead, use serum, your powerhouse potent product that will deliver the maximum benefits with its high absorption rate. Serum doesn't sit on the surface and protect your skin, it penetrates and really makes a difference. You can start using it in your twenties as your targeted treatment; in your thirties and forties, use a serum with anti-aging benefits.

Make sure you treat the neck and décolletage with the same cleanser, exfoliator, serum, and moisturizer as the rest of the face. Don't forget the back of the neck and behind the ears, either. After all, that's the area that is cut into to lift and remove the slackening during a facelift.

A NOTE ON HANDS

One of the great age giveaways, hands are exposed all the time yet often neglected. Hydration and UV protection are essential to keep the skin healthy and supple and free from age spots.

\# Be conscious about how often you wash your hands and reapply moisturizer afterward.

\# Keep a tube of hand cream in your purse, on your desk, by the bed, and next to the sink.

\# If your hands are really dry, apply a treatment oil and wear softening gloves overnight.

\# If you drive a lot, wear gloves (thin cotton ones won't be too hot in the summer)—your hands are right up there by the windshield and UV rays can penetrate glass.

Top tip Don't forget to look after your eyelids and keep them moisturized. They have to stretch over the eyeballs constantly and, as we get older, the skin loses its elasticity, resulting in saggy eyes. If an eye cream, gel, or serum feels sticky and heavy on the lids, use it as a mask—leave it to sink in for 10 minutes and then gently pat off the excess—or just put it on at night.

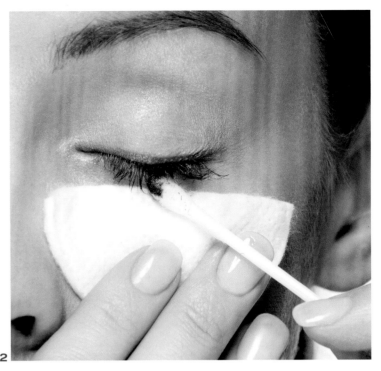

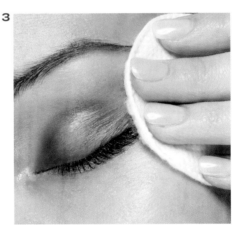

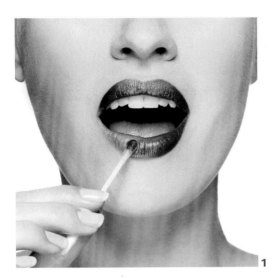

1 To remove lipstick, dip a Q-tip in make-up remover and gently rub it over your lips. **2** Stubborn mascara or eyeliner can be removed using a Q-tip, too. First fold a cotton pad in half and place the flat edge under your lower lashes. Dip the Q-tip in oil-based eye-make-up remover, close your eye and stroke it over your lashes and lash line. **3** Soak a cotton pad in eye-make-up remover. Hold it over your closed eye for 30 seconds, then gently wipe the make-up away—don't scrub or rub the eyes.

Morning & evening

1 Cleanse your face, neck, and décolletage thoroughly. If you only do this once a day, make sure it's in the evening, to remove all the dirt, grime, sweat, and sebum.

2 Apply a targeted eye serum or cream.

3 Apply a treatment serum—this could be anti-aging, hydrating, balancing, radiance-boosting, or pigment-correcting.

4 In the morning, apply protective daily moisturizer with SPF. At night, apply a treatment oil and lashings of hand cream (see opposite).

5 If you wish, apply a separate neck and décolletage cream.

Don't forget your body—exfoliate in the shower and always moisturize your body, too.

FACIAL MASSAGE

Facial massage is a great way to release tension and give skin a lifting boost. Massage techniques can be used on dry skin in need of a pick-me-up, or as part of your cleansing regime for an ultradraining and blockage-clearing treatment—it will help to boost the absorption of creams and serums and maximize their results.

Create a **LOOSE FIST** with your palms facing your chin and use your knuckles to massage product all over your face, working from the center out toward your ears and down the sides of the neck. Focus on your chin, jaw, and lower face. To de-clog your pores, work in an upward direction with your fingertips and encourage drainage by working toward the lymph nodes just under the earlobes.

Use the **FLAT AND HEEL OF YOUR THUMB** and the side of your bent forefinger in a pinching flick movement along your jawline from chin to ear.

Using your fingertips, move in a **ROTARY MOTION** all over your face from the center outward, from chin to ear, upper lip to ear, nose to temple, and along the brow and forehead.

Use your fingertips to **TAP OVER YOUR SKIN**, gently drumming on either side of your face. Applying eye serum in this way helps to de-puff the area and drain excess fluid.

Use the flat of your hands to **GENTLY STROKE UPWARD** from your brow across your forehead to ease tension and lift the skin. Use the same technique on your neck, stroking in an upward motion from chest to chin.

Use the **TIPS OF YOUR FOREFINGERS** on pressure points all over your face—stimulating these areas helps to energize the skin, de-puff, and stimulate lymphatic drainage.

MASSAGE AROUND THE EYE CONTOURS to help brighten the eye area and drain any fluid build-up. Start on one side of the nose and work your way around the eye using small circular motions and light pressure with your fingertips.

FINISH BY PINCHING your earlobes between your thumb and forefinger.

It is a good sign if your skin has a pink flush. This means you have increased blood circulation, which in turn oxygenates and feeds cells, and helps drain cellular waste, giving you a post-facial glow.

TOP TIPS FOR HEALTHY SKIN

\# Cut down on sugar and caffeine, which cause cell destruction, collagen breakdown, and slackening of the skin, as well as being very dehydrating. If you can't avoid them altogether, counteract their negative effects by detoxing when you need to with a five-day juice diet and drinking at least 8 glasses (2 litres) of water a day.

\# Carry water with you all the time to make it easy to stay hydrated. Choose still over carbonated, as the bubbles contribute to cellulite and bloating. Get a portable water "bobble," a bottle that has a built-in carbon filter. Every time you feel thirsty, so does your skin: if your lips, eyes, or mouth feel dry, your skin does, too.

\# A daily supplement of omega oils helps keep skin healthy and resilient.

\# Use UV protection every day and reapply it regularly.

\# Self-massage using a facial oil improves the general functioning of the skin and helps relieve line-causing tension. Massage boosts the circulation, which feeds cells with nutrients and oxygen, and helps lymph drainage, the body's way of removing toxins and waste.

The 5 greatest skin concerns

These are the most common problems or worries about skin that Sarah Chapman encounters in her salon.

1

Is there a way to erase pigmentation?

I see pigmentation a lot and it's very hard to get rid off. A course of IPL (intense pulsed light) or laser treatments are usually the most effective. Daily use of a pigment-controlling serum and UV protection are absolutely key to prevent further damage.

2

Why have I got adult acne?

Far from being an exclusively teenage concern, acne and breakouts are usually hormone-related or stress-induced and often affect people in their forties. This can be distressing, especially for people who never had spots as a teenager, and there is the additional challenge of trying to combat aging along with treating pimples. Mild peels work well, as they help smooth lines as well as controlling breakouts. The use of Retinol will also address both problems.

3

What can I do about my slackening skin?

Where Botox used to be the go-to treatment to iron out wrinkles, increasingly loss of volume and slackening skin is the greater concern. The daily use of products that stimulate dermal collagen production, such as peptides and stem cells, will help to improve the "bounce" of the skin. Alternatively, certain laser treatments or fillers can be used to plump and create volume.

4

How can I combat dullness and lack of radiance?

The best way to achieve a healthy glow is to adopt a good skin-maintenance routine, making sure you exfoliate regularly to lift off dull dead cells and keep hydration levels high. A good facial will give you these results instantly.

5

How can I reduce my skin's sensitivity and redness

A reaction can be triggered by the incorrect use of products or treatments, such as too much dermabrasion, or it can be due to underlying cellular inflammation. Treat the skin with care and support it with supplements and products that will boost the immune function. Make sure you keep the skin protected.

beauty
first aid

There are certain
beauty concerns
that I come across
time and time again,
many of which are
very simple to remedy
with the right products
and techniques.

**This troubleshooting section tackles
some of the most frequently fretted-over
problems—such as eye bags, dark circles,
blemishes, and age spots—and shows
you simple ways to conceal or disguise
them. If your beauty concern relates to
a skin condition, do consider whether
there is an underlying cause that needs
to be addressed, such as your diet,
lifestyle, or a reaction to skincare
products or cosmetics.**

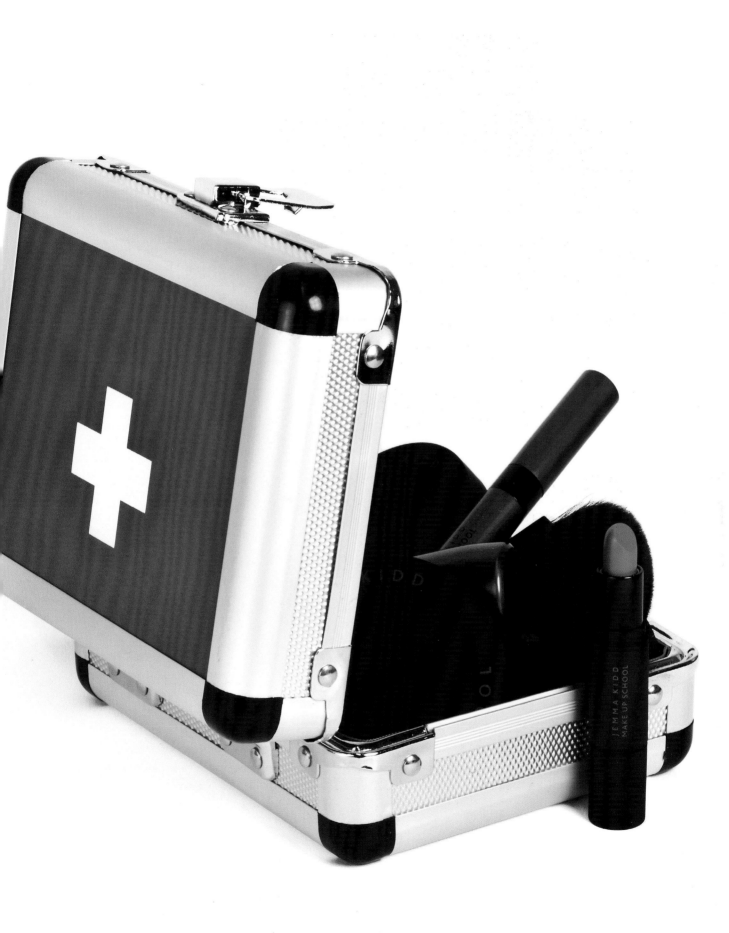

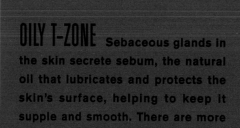

OILY T-ZONE
Sebaceous glands in the skin secrete sebum, the natural oil that lubricates and protects the skin's surface, helping to keep it supple and smooth. There are more sebaceous glands in the T-zone than in the cheeks, and overactive glands result in a shiny forehead, nose, and chin due to excess sebum. This often leads to clogged pores and breakouts, and makes it harder for make-up to stay in place. The most important thing is to cleanse morning and night with a suitable nonstripping oil-based cleanser, and then moisturize, as oily skin is often dehydrated (see pages 158 and 171). Think about your diet, too, as there are often simple adjustments that you can make to balance your skin (see pages 162–7). There are good primers and foundations for oily skin, which control shine and keep it matte. Using a mattifying primer under foundation will help it stay in place and means you can use less, reducing the risk of clogged pores. Silica helps to absorb oil and keep it locked away from the skin's surface, so look for it in primer, foundation, and powder. Mineral powder foundation is perfect for oily skin, as the oil helps the powder to be absorbed, giving a natural finish. Alternatively, use a light foundation and buff your skin with fine loose powder. To avoid powder build-up on oily skin, use an oil-blotting paper before touching up make-up. Be aware that wax-based cream blushes, bronzers, and eyeshadows may slide off oily skin.

DRY PATCHES
Dry skin often feels tight and may result in flaky patches. Possible causes are dehydration, poor diet, stress, overexposure to the sun or cold, or a reaction to skincare products or cosmetics. On-going symptoms could be due to a condition such as eczema or psoriasis, so see your doctor if this is the case. Always choose hydrating formulas and exfoliate regularly to remove dead surface skin.

Make-up sits on the surface of dry skin, so massage your face with a hydrating serum or oil before moisturizing. A light liquid foundation will work better for you than cream or stick formulas. Oil-based products will glide on easily, whereas powder products tend to sit in creases and draw attention to lines and flakiness. Cream blush is preferable to powder blush for this reason.

DULL, LACKLUSTER SKIN
Skin can look dull when you are tired, stressed, or not eating well or drinking enough water. Use a gentle skin-brightening exfoliator to reveal fresh, new skin. Treat the face to a radiance-boosting mask and stimulate the circulation with massage (see page 174). Use a hydrating moisturizer to keep the skin looking dewy and supple, so it naturally reflects the light.

Choose light-reflecting formulas for your primer, foundation, and powder, and add a separate illuminator to your foundation. Sheer or soft pearl finishes and cream textures reflect the light, so avoid anything too matte. Finish your make-up by using a highlighter or radiance cream on the raised areas of your face that would naturally catch the light (see pages 26–7).

Before

Above Red indicates the area that should be shaded (see right). Blue shows where the highlighter should be applied. Blend it along the cheekbones and add a touch to the chin and bow of the mouth to catch the light and draw attention to those areas. Remember, you need to blend and blend and blend when you're doing any kind of contouring or shaping.

STRONG JAW

Clever shading can minimize the appearance of a heavy or square jawline. Dark colors make an area recede (see pages 26–7), so choose a matte powder or a cream product or foundation that is no more than two shades darker than the natural skin tone. You are not brightening or warming the skin, you are creating shadow, so the color should be flat with grayish undertones—what I call "dead" or "non-" colors—and the payoff has to be weak, because it's all about layering and creating a real softness. Begin the shading level with the middle of the ear and bring it down and around the jaw, to about halfway to your chin, depending on your face. Shade the color from underneath the jawbone, so it fades in and up to the face and blends down onto the neck and up onto the temples.

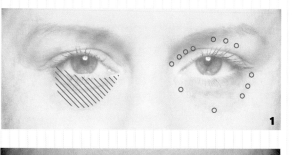

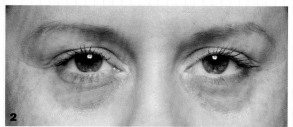

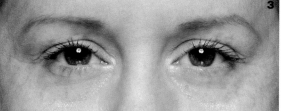

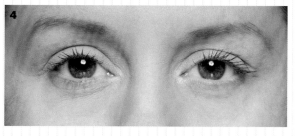

DARK CIRCLES
Lack of sleep and dehydration make dark circles a common problem (2). The aim is to conceal them without making the skin cakey. First apply my Citrus Color Corrector (see page 25), dabbing it on with your finger or a concealer brush and gently pressing it into the skin. This counteracts the red, blue, and purple undertones (see the red shaded area, 1). Then apply apricot color corrector on top to warm up the skin for a natural daytime look (3). For the evening, you may want to add more coverage (4). If you have just applied color correctors, let them "set" into the skin for a few minutes, then apply a little creamy concealer the same color as the skin on top (see the blue dotted area, 1). Apply foundation to the rest of the face and set with fine translucent powder. Use an eye primer, such as my I-Perfector, over the eyelid and on the inner rims to neutralize any redness and brighten the eyes.

FEATHERING AROUND THE LIPS
This is when lipstick, stain, or gloss "bleeds" beyond the lip line and settles into the fine lines around the mouth. It becomes a common problem with age, as the lips become drier, less plump, and more wrinkled. Oily and liquid formulas travel more: thicker and drier formulas are more likely to stay put.
Prep the mouth with primer and a light dusting of powder. Outline the lips with lip liner to create a waxy barrier. The brighter the color, the more obvious the bleed, so use a neutral liner. Draw the outline, smile to stretch your lips, and reapply. Use a lip brush to apply lipstick with greater precision and blot with a tissue, then brush a little powder around the lips to seal in the color. Keep gloss to the middle part of the lips, away from the edges.

CHAPPED LIPS
The skin on the lips is thin and lacks glands that produce the natural oils that keep skin smooth and protected. As a result, lips dry out faster and become chapped more easily when you are dehydrated or exposed to extreme temperatures, so keep fluid levels topped up and apply balm to moisturize and protect the lips. Always choose moisturizing lipsticks and glosses.
To smooth away dry, flaky skin, apply lip scrub or balm, and rub the lips gently back and forth using a Q-tip, soft toothbrush, or washcloth. Wipe the lips clean and apply a generous coat of lip balm containing natural oils, such as beeswax or shea butter, and SPF to protect the lips from harmful UV rays. Reapply regularly, especially after eating or drinking. (See also pages 88–9.)

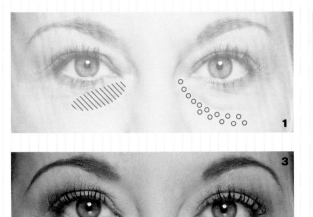

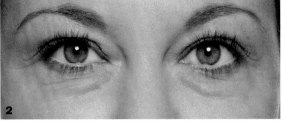

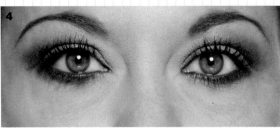

EYE BAGS

A build-up of toxins and fluid retention in the undereye tissue results in puffiness. As well as being aging, the protrusion creates dark shadows that make the eyes look heavy and tired (2). Bags become more noticeable with age, due to the loss of elasticity and collagen.

A cool compress can reduce inflammation, but the technique for concealing eye bags involves shading and highlighting. First, apply a creamy concealer or full-coverage foundation one shade darker than your skin tone to the puffy area (see the red shading, 1) to make it recede. Then apply a highlighter to the indent (see the blue dotted area, 1) to bring it forward. The contrast will be obvious, so blend a skin-brightening soft pearl apricot powder over the eye area to flatten it and make it look more two-dimensional. Enhance the eyes with a soft smoky look for day (3), adding more drama for night (4). This will create a lifting effect and makes the eyes look larger.

AGE SPOTS

With age, melanin, the pigment that protects the skin from sun damage, can clump together to form brown liver spots, so always wear high-factor sunscreen on exposed areas of the skin to minimize the risk of age spots forming.

To reduce their appearance, apply moisturizer with SPF followed by primer to create a smooth base, then use a peach-colored concealer, which helps to cancel out the darkness of age spots. Dab a little onto the age spot with your ring finger, which has the lightest touch so ensures you can build up the product gradually. Tap your finger over the age spot until it is covered and then lightly sweep a small brush over the concealer to create a more natural texture. Apply foundation on top to blend the concealer into the skin and make it less noticeable. Dust the face with powder to create an even tone and set the make-up. For fuller coverage, use a product such as Dermablend (see Moles, page 182). Age spots around the mouth can change the shape of the lips, so use my Lip Perfector to conceal them and create a sharp neutral outline (see left).

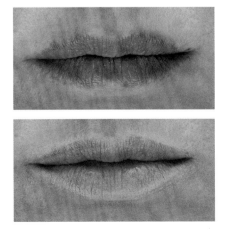

ACNE

For a long-term solution, do consult a dermatologist, who can prescribe the correct course of treatment, and look at your diet (see page 164). In the short term, the right make-up can cover your blemishes and make your skin look flawless and radiant.

Good hygiene helps to prevent the spread of acne-causing bacteria, so store cosmetics in a cool, dry place and wash brushes and sponges regularly. Always wash your hands and use an acne-fighting cleanser before applying make-up. A good tip is to apply Visine eye drops with a Q-tip or cotton pad to take out some of the redness.

Apply primer—if your skin has red patches, try a tinted primer that contains a color corrector—then blend a light, oil-free foundation evenly over your face. Blemishes and pimples that are still visible need to be covered with a concealer—Laura Mercier Secret Camouflage is a good choice, because it is very dense and gives full coverage. If you need to tone down redness, use my Citrus Color Corrector first, then choose a concealer that matches your skin tone and dab it over the pimples, blending the edges carefully. Set with ultrafine loose powder for long-lasting coverage.

SPOTS

Don't be tempted to squeeze a spot, as this could lead to inflammation or infection. Treat it with an antibacterial solution to help speed up healing—I like to use Tea Tree Oil or Witch Hazel to dry out spots.

Cover the spot with a firm but creamy yellow-toned concealer—nothing that dries to a flaky finish, which will draw attention to it. Lightly tap the concealer in place with a clean finger or brush, and then blend it out at the edges, taking care not to wipe it off. Apply foundation carefully, covering the blended edges of the concealer. When it has absorbed, set with fine powder—I like apricot-toned powder because it brightens the skin. If you need to retouch the spot, wash your hands, apply another dab of concealer and blend as before, then re-set with powder.

MOLES

SPF is really important to protect moles from sun damage. To conceal a mole, prep and prime the skin in the usual way. A pale mole might be covered adequately using foundation and concealer, but be careful—products that are too light will make a mole look ashy, and if it is raised, it may end up looking more like a pimple. For dark moles, try a fuller "camouflage" coverage such as Dermablend. This is a very thick product, which you should warm in the palm of your hand before applying. Gently push it into the skin with your ring finger, allow it to dry, then reapply if necessary, and set with fine translucent powder. On the hole, moles are very difficult to hide, so try to learn to love your mole.

RED SPOTS

Prep and prime the skin as usual and apply foundation, which should tone down any redness. Then use my Citrus Color Corrector to cover red spots. Dab it onto the center of the spot with a brush and blend it gently. Choose a concealer that matches your skin tone and apply a little over the color corrector to make it less noticeable. Finish with a dusting of fine translucent powder to set.

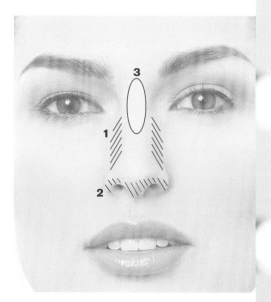

1 Apply subtle shading down both sides of the nose to narrow the bridge, blending it well and making sure it is symmetrical.

2 Shade the underside of the tip of the nose to give the illusion that it is shorter than it is and the nostrils are less bulbous.

3 Blend a little highlighter down the top part of the bridge of the nose, taking care not to take it down the sides. This will catch the light and bring that area forward.

STRONG NOSE If you are worried that your nose is too prominent, there are ways to minimize its impact without succumbing to the surgeon's knife. As with all contouring and shading, the effect must be incredibly subtle and soft so that it looks really natural (see pages 26–7). Use a shade of foundation or a matte cream or powder contouring product slightly darker than your skin to create the shadow. Apply a line down both sides of the bridge of your nose, positioning them to create the desired width. Then blend really well, making sure the result is symmetrical. If you want to create the illusion of a shorter nose, apply the same color to the base of the tip, again blending it really well. Highlight the top of the bridge to catch the light.

holding back the years

As we get older, most of us have a few typical beauty complaints associated with the aging process. When those first signs begin to appear, there's no need to go for extreme solutions—there is a lot you can do with your skincare regime and make-up to keep you looking younger for longer.

There are several factors that contribute to the overall changes we face. Skin cells don't rejuvenate as fast as they did and, as it thins, skin starts to loose its luminosity and dehydrates more easily. Less collagen and elastin are produced and without these supporting tissues the skin becomes less plump, and fine lines and wrinkles begin to make a few changes around the eyes and lips in particular. Hair follicles shrink, so hair becomes thinner, and brows and lashes may get sparser as a result. In addition, the skin cells that produce melanin on exposure to UV rays can overproduce the pigment, causing the appearance of age spots.

Don't despair—being aware of why these changes take place is the first step to slowing them down.

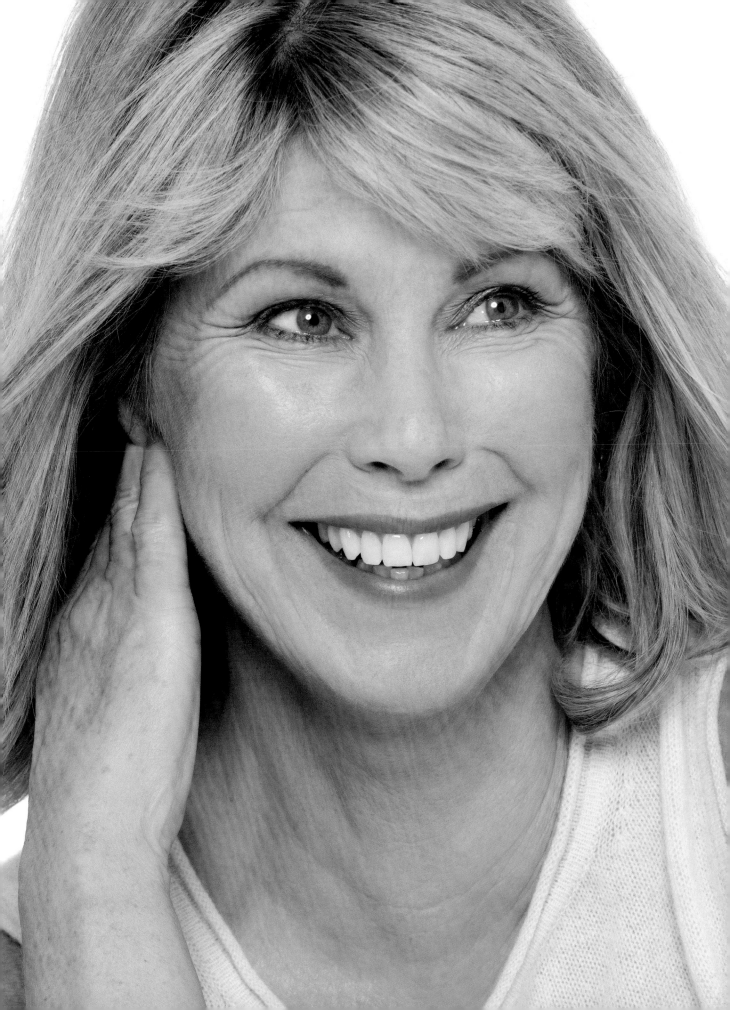

SKIN SENSE THROUGH THE AGES

Your skin will change as you age, so how you treat it when you are in your forties and beyond should be different from when you were in your teens and twenties.

Not everybody is the same. Sometimes women in their forties have skin that looks ten years younger than their age, whereas others in their thirties have the skin of someone ten years older. So look at the condition of your own skin and don't be afraid to use products that you didn't feel were "meant" for you.

how old is your skin?

Try these quick tests to help you assess how advanced your signs of aging are.

SLACKENING SKIN

Place a mirror flat on a table in front of you and look down at yourself. Anywhere on your face that is losing its tone and volume will drop downward. This gives you a good indication of what your face is going to look like as it changes over the years.

DEEP LINES

Keep your face expressionless and look in the mirror. Any lines that are there when your face is static, and don't just appear when you are smiling and frowning, are set. You can soften the appearance of these lines by keeping the skin as healthy, relaxed, and moisturized as possible—regular facials improve the skin's tone and texture—but the only things that will remove deep lines altogether are Botox or fillers.

LINES AROUND THE MOUTH

The skin around the mouth changes as we get older, leading to feathering and then deeper lines and less-full lips. This is mainly due to a change in hormone levels and decreasing estrogen, but also because it is an area that is constantly moving. Keep the skin hydrated and try toning up the muscles with facial exercises. If your thinning lips really bother you, as they do a lot of women, consider having a filler, but don't do anything too extreme, as it can look so unnatural.

treatments to turn back time

There are many procedures and treatments available, but I have personally seen positive results with these. Possible side effects are well documented, so my advice is to always do your research thoroughly and, if possible, go with a personal recommendation. Always remember, too, moderation is key—do it little and often and only when you really feel you need it.

Botox These wrinkle-relaxing injections are proven to reduce frown lines and crow's feet, and can help prevent new lines from forming. The effects last around three months.

Dermal fillers Injectable fillers such as Restylane® are effective in reducing facial lines and smoothing out pronounced wrinkles, such as nose-to-mouth grooves, deep forehead furrows, and crow's feet. They are also used to restore plumpness to lips and cheeks, reversing the sunken or jowly look. This is an instant "lunch-hour" treatment, but do insist on a subtle result, as fillers can look really artificial if they are not done in moderation.

Chemical peels This sounds drastic, but there are varying concentrations depending on your needs. Chemical peels can be used to treat problems such as sun damage, hyperpigmentation, tired-looking skin caused by a build-up of dead cells, fine lines, and wrinkles. After treatment, skin appears softer, regenerated, and more uniform. If you find the term "chemical" off-putting, Mother Nature does her own version—papaya, pumpkin, and pineapple extracts are all rich in natural AHAs (Alpha Hydroxy Acids) and do a similar job very naturally.

IPL (Intense Pulsed Light) A course of IPL rejuvenating therapy stimulates collagen production and improves the skin's elasticity and overall color and texture. It is a good treatment for rosacea, thread veins, broken capillaries, sun damage, and age spots. I've tried this one myself and it really worked.

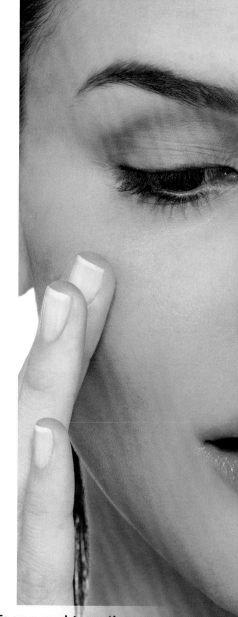

Teens and twenties
When you are younger, you probably need lighter formulations with less of the core anti-aging ingredients. SPF is essential to prevent damage that will age the skin faster.

Thirties and forties
Skin begins to show signs of any damage done during your teens and twenties, so now is the time to step up the anti-aging repair.

Fifties, sixties, and beyond
These are the decades when the huge shift in hormones will change the skin significantly and you also need to deal with hot flashes, sensitivity, and dryness—the average age of menopause is 52.

Many of today's multitasking make-up formulations are rich in anti-aging ingredients. These help to repair and protect your skin from further damage, while improving its texture and tone and adding youthful color to your face.

Aside from the dreaded wrinkles, one of the telltale signs of an aging face is the dull, lackluster quality of the skin. What's missing is that fresh, radiant glow of youthful health. Skin brighteners are key to putting this right, but nothing too metallic or silver; it needs that warmth—the apricot and soft gold tones with a lightly pearlized finish that help to bring dull skin alive and make it softly luminous.

MAKE-UP TO MAKE YOU
LOOK YOUNGER

HELPFUL HINTS

As older skin is thinner, it tends to dry out easily and become less supple and papery, so protecting it from cold winds and low temperatures is just as important as shielding it from UV rays.

If you have bad sun damage or thread veins, there are treatments (such as IPL, see page 187) that will lessen and even reverse the damage. I think it is well worth having these done.

Use pencil and/or powder to define your eyebrows and lash line to frame your face. Working brown eyeliner into the roots of the lashes gives the illusion of thicker, more abundant lashes.

Be careful to blend products really well to make sure that nothing settles in the fine lines or draws attention to wrinkles.

If your eyesight isn't what it was, use a magnifying mirror and always work in good light.

GOLDEN RULE

Always think: nothing too light, bright, or shimmery, and nothing too dark and hard.

color

Concentrate on creating softness and warmth. Stay away from black and gray as you grow older—dark brown eyeliner and lash tint will be much less harsh than black. Go with softer colors and tones that help to brighten up the skin—apricot, peach, and warm browns are flattering to all skin tones.

For lipsticks, it is best to stick within the mid-tones and go for the shades that are closest to your natural lip color.

textures

With age, you have to work harder at keeping skin hydrated and plump like a ripe fruit. It will depend on your skin's natural tendency, but the majority of time skin becomes drier as you get older, rather than oilier, so a light hydrating cream foundation is ideal.

As a rule, try to use less product on your skin; so if you have sun spots and discoloration, use a color corrector to address this but keep your application of foundation and powder as minimal as possible. Sometimes it is worth consulting a dermatologist to get sun spots and thread veins seen to. I'm all for this, as then you need less coverage, which is less masking.

Stains and cream blushes both work well on older skin. A sheer stain mimics that youthful flush, and a cream is hydrating and natural-looking—go for a mousse or cream-to-powder finish that is neither too wet and greasy nor too cakey on the skin.

Avoid metallic finishes, which tend to highlight lines and crepiness, and stay away from liquid eyeliners and hard lines. Use a creamy eye pencil to define the eyes, with a little eyeshadow in the same color dabbed on top to make it last longer and look softer. Eyes often water more as you get older, so lash tint can work well, giving natural-looking definition.

As lips tend to lose their plumpness, strong matte lipsticks can be aging and accentuate thinness. Instead, go for creamy textures that are hydrating and nourishing. Use a neutral shade mixed with balm or layered with gloss to make lips look fuller. Lip stains bring that lovely youthful red-wine color back to your mouth—the natural berry red of a child's lips—but if you use a liquid formula, take care that it doesn't "bleed." A waxy lip liner in a nude shade becomes a make-up bag must-have to seal in color.

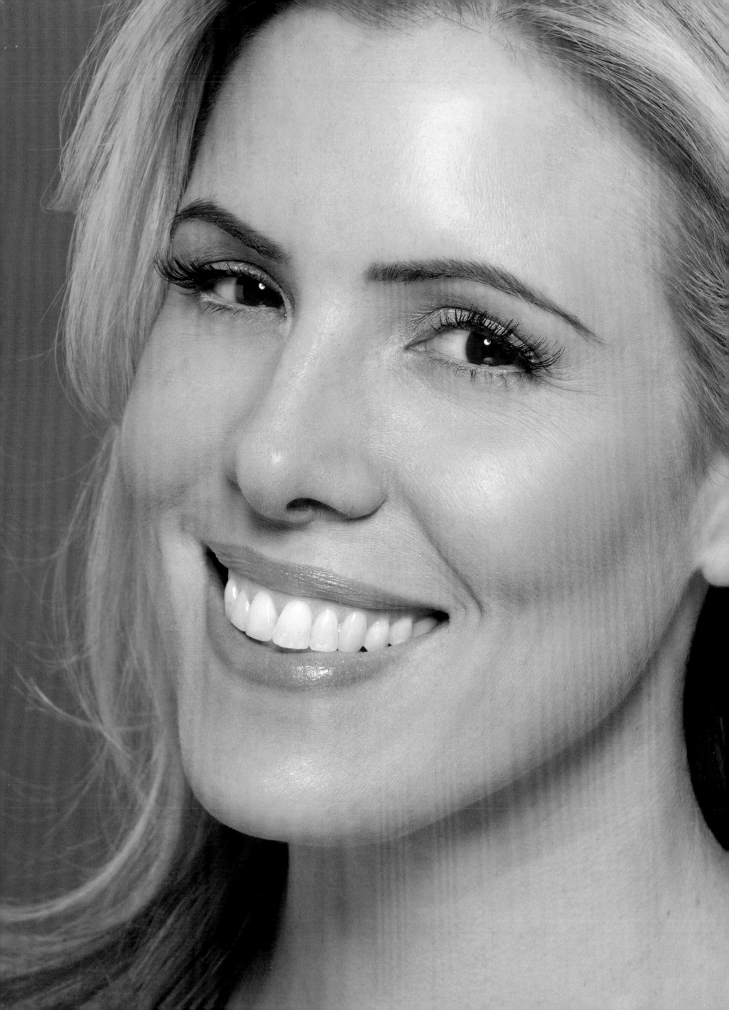

Forties

The skin is the biggest indicator of how young you look, so make it look amazing. The pinky peach of the eye, lip, and blush colors blend together well, so that nothing deflects from the youthful radiance that takes years off.

Eyes

The make-up palette is very natural, so make the brows slightly darker than usual to frame and structure the face.

Use an eye primer to neutralize any redness, which can be very aging.

All the focus is on the skin, so keep the eyes understated with a simple wash of peach-toned nude powder eyeshadow (1) over the lid.

Curl the lashes and apply black mascara. Then add corner lashes to open up and elongate the eyes.

Skin

The older we get, the skin becomes more pigmented, and fine capillaries and thread veins often show more, so use a medium-coverage foundation and concealer where you need it, especially around the nose and under the eyes. To bring out your skin's radiance, mix a little cream highlighter (2) with the foundation on the back of your hand. This gives the skin a soft luminosity rather than an obvious highlight.

Dust the T-zone lightly with mineral powder to set the make-up.

Cheeks loose their plumpness as we age, so use blush (3) to emphasize the pillowy apples of the cheeks. Peach tones are incredibly flattering on most skin tones, being neither too pink nor too orange. Pink can be too youthful, but peach has a maturity to it and matches skin tones better. Brush it along the cheekbones and blend it into the apples of the cheeks to bring out a natural-looking flush and warm up the face.

Lips

Apply a moisturizing creamy lipstick with a shiny finish in a peachy shade (4), so there are no clashing colors.

Skincare expert Sarah Chapman's top five tips for younger-looking skin

Monthly facials I am a big believer in making a professional facial a regular part of a skincare regime, as I've seen at first hand the difference it makes. Ladies who have done this for years undoubtedly have stronger, more resilient skin that looks younger and healthier than those who haven't.

Facial massage Regular massage of the face, neck, and décolletage, as part of a treatment or at home (see page 174), is a great way to keep the skin supple, radiant, and in good condition.

Peels If you have oily, dull, problematic, sun-damaged, or thickened skin, I recommend having a course of mild peels. However, if you have thin skin, avoid microdermabrasion, a deep exfoliating treatment that removes the protective epidermis and thins the skin, which is what the aging process does anyway; it can make the skin more prone to pigmentation damage.

Cocktailing I'm not suggesting you overdo the Cosmopolitans, I'm talking about your products. Add a little extra-concentrated, treatment product to your moisturizer or facial oil. If you don't have time to apply serum, moisturizer, and SPF, for example, just mix a bit of everything in your palm and put it on.

Use an occlusive mask Made from alginate, which turns rubbery when applied to the face, occlusive masks help serum to penetrate the skin. Apply serum and use the mask to maximize its effect.

Sixties

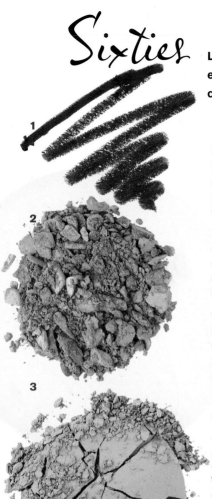

Less is more when it comes to make-up in your sixties, as you don't want to emphasize fine lines and wrinkles. The focus is on bringing a little youthful color back to the face and making brows, lashes, and lips look fuller.

Eyes

Blend eye primer over the lids to neutralize redness and use a nude eye pencil along the inner rims to open up the eyes and make them look bigger.

Brush natural powder through the eyebrows to make them look fuller by creating a shadow by the roots. Apply a little at a time using an angled brow brush and blend it out, then repeat.

With a dark brown eye pencil (1), which is more flattering and easier to wear than black, work between the roots of lashes to make them look thicker and give the eyes subtle definition.

Blend a warm taupe eyeshadow (2) over the lid for a neutral wash of color.

Curl the lashes and apply black mascara. If your eyes are prone to watering, use a waterproof lash tint on the bottom lashes. Add corner lashes to enhance and open up the eyes.

Skin

Color correctors come into their own, as they are very sheer and cover imperfections without loading the skin with product and emphasizing wrinkles. Brighten up the skin beneath the eyes with an apricot-toned color corrector.

Apply primer (3) for a smooth base, then dot foundation only on areas that need it, and blend well so that it doesn't settle in the fine lines. Make sure no redness or blemishes come through.

Brighten the cheekbones with a light dusting of illuminating powder and blend peach blush (4) over the apples of the cheeks to create a natural flush.

Lips

Pat lip primer over the lips and outline them with a waxy pencil to conceal pigmentation and prevent feathering.

Using your finger or a lip brush, pat a sheer berry color (5) over the lips. This gives lighter coverage than if you apply it straight from the tube, more like a stain. The finish is natural because the texture of the lips shows though.

OVER 50: DOS AND DON'TS

Do

Choose colors that look natural against your skin; stick with rose- or coral-toned lipstick or gloss. Use peachy blush: smile and apply it to the apples of your cheeks, then blend, blend, blend. Use mascara or lash tint, but sparingly on the lower lashes; use waterproof if your eyes water. Apply light-reflecting foundation or tinted moisturizer, but only where you really need it. Blend creamy concealer with moisturizer to ensure that it doesn't cake or settle in fine lines.

Don't

Wear vibrant, contrasting, or strong, hard colors. Use metallic or shimmer make-up, as it exaggerates the texture of the skin and draws attention to lines and crepiness. Choose flat matte products, especially matte lipstick, as it makes the lips look thin and lifeless. Apply blush to the bones of the cheeks—with age, cheeks often become sunken, and applying blush to the bones exaggerates any hollowness and makes us look gaunt.

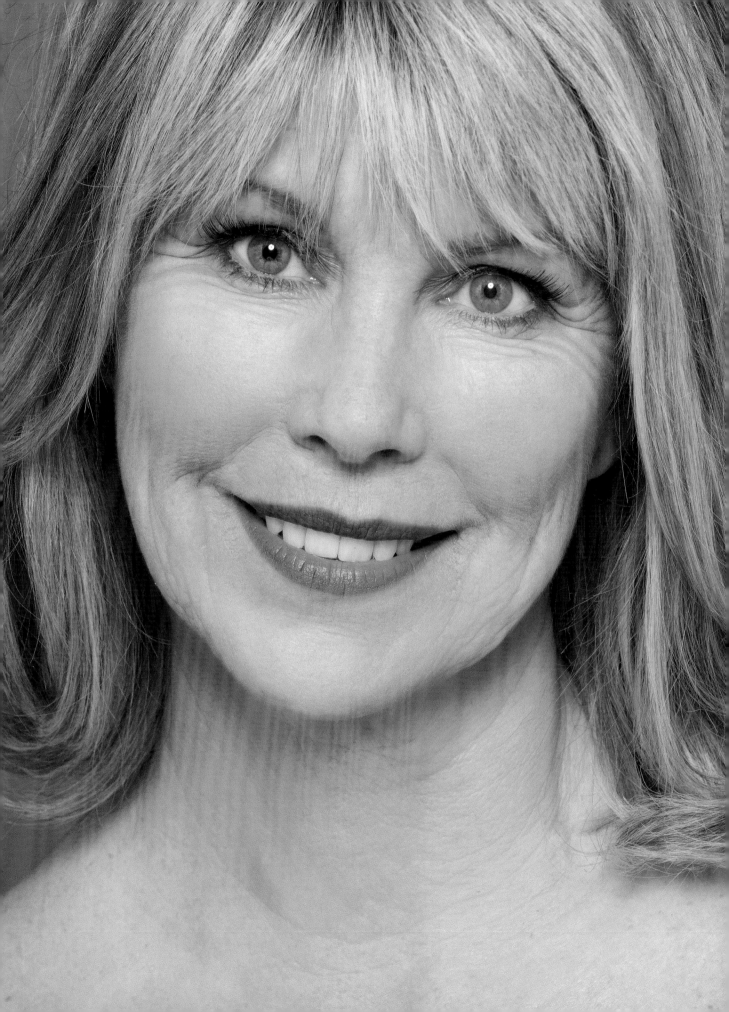

Top 10 tips for youthful skin

1

The outer layer of the skin becomes thinner, cells divide more slowly, and dead skin cells do not shed as easily, so use a gentle exfoliator and then apply a nourishing moisturizer to optimize the skin's condition.

2

Massage a facial oil into the skin regularly to keep it supple, restore its elasticity, and aid circulation.

3

Skin repairs itself at night while you sleep, so make sure you get eight hours' rest a night and use a serum and a rich, moisturizing night cream that stimulates cell regeneration.

4

In addition to the all-round benefits to your health and wellbeing, taking regular exercise increases circulation, so more nutrients are carried to the skin which helps promote the renewal of skin cells.

5

Watch what you eat. Excess sugar, alcohol, and caffeine can accelerate the aging process. Foods that are high in antioxidants help to protect the skin. I drink cucumber juice and eat raw vegetables every day for the minerals and enzymes.

6

Essential fatty acids are fantastic for the skin, as well as for the hair, nails, and general health—Udo's Choice Oil is beauty in a bottle.

7

Avoid heavy foundation and instead use a color corrector and concealer, if you need to, and add soft luminosity to the face with light-reflecting tinted moisturizer or radiance cream—BB creams are fantastic.

8

Stay away from matte or powdery make-up, as a dry, flat finish will emphasize wrinkles and fine lines. Shiny metallic or highlighting products will also draw attention to areas that you would rather play down.

9

Pink or peach cream blush on the apples of the cheeks has a brightening effect and restores a youthful flush. If you have oil-control problems, choose a fine skin-brightening powder and use a large, soft brush to "polish" the skin and ensure it doesn't settle in the fine lines.

10

Remove your make-up every night without fail. Keep a pack of cleansing wipes by your bed, so there is never an excuse to sleep in your make-up.

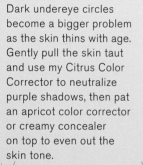

Top 10 tips for beautiful eyes and lips

1

Sensitive thin skin around the eyes is most prone to lines, so invest in a dedicated anti-aging eye serum.

2

Wear sunglasses on sunny days all year round. Not only will they help protect you from the sun's rays, but squinting less will help to prevent crow's feet and frown lines.

3

Dark undereye circles become a bigger problem as the skin thins with age. Gently pull the skin taut and use my Citrus Color Corrector to neutralize purple shadows, then pat an apricot color corrector or creamy concealer on top to even out the skin tone.

4

Apply dark brown pencil eyeliner at the roots of the lashes and then go over it with a dark powder eyeshadow and smudge the line gently. This gives a much better illusion of thick lashes than extra mascara.

5

Opt for soft shades of brown or gray, especially for eyeliner, as black can be too harsh. You can still wear black mascara, but don't apply it too thickly.

6

Keep your eyebrows neat, but be sure not to overpluck. Fill in any sparse areas with an eyebrow pencil and go over it with powder the same shade as your hair to make the brows look fuller and natural.

7

Fine lines around the mouth mean that lipstick will "bleed" unless you use a waxy lip liner. Draw the outline first, then smile to stretch your lips and reapply. Brush a little translucent powder around the lip line to seal in the color.

8

Give up the strong, matte lipsticks and use soft pink, peach, or nude shades in moisturizing, nourishing formulations that will keep lips hydrated and plumped.

9

Try mixing your lipstick with a waxy balm, or layer it with a little light gloss to keep lips supple and make them look fuller.

10

A good trick is to apply lipstick with your finger, pressing it into the lip to give a stainlike finish. This method allows you to wear stronger colors, as the effect is more sheer and natural-looking.

seasonal shift

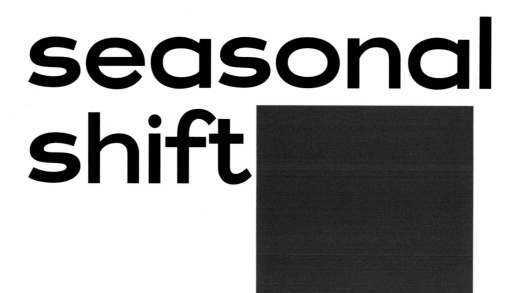

Think about your make-up in the same way as your clothes and overhaul your cosmetics bag, along with your closet, every time the seasons change.

When the nights draw in and the air starts to bite, we automatically reach for our cozy knits and warm coats, and when the days lengthen and we feel the sun's warmth, we're pleased to swap them for floaty florals and crisp cottons. For make-up, too, a shift in color palette is natural. In the summer we tend to be drawn to vibrant colors or pretty pastels and sheer, light textures, while winter calls for darker shades and velvety soft or rich creamy finishes.

With a change in climate there often comes a change to your skin, and this also needs to be taken into account in terms of the products you use. Summer demands greater protection from UV rays, and intense heat can cause the skin to produce more oil and sweat. In winter, cold wind and central heating often cause dry patches and redness, which call for rich products that hydrate, protect, and comfort.

Take this opportunity to sort through your make-up and throw away any old, unused, or out-of-date products.

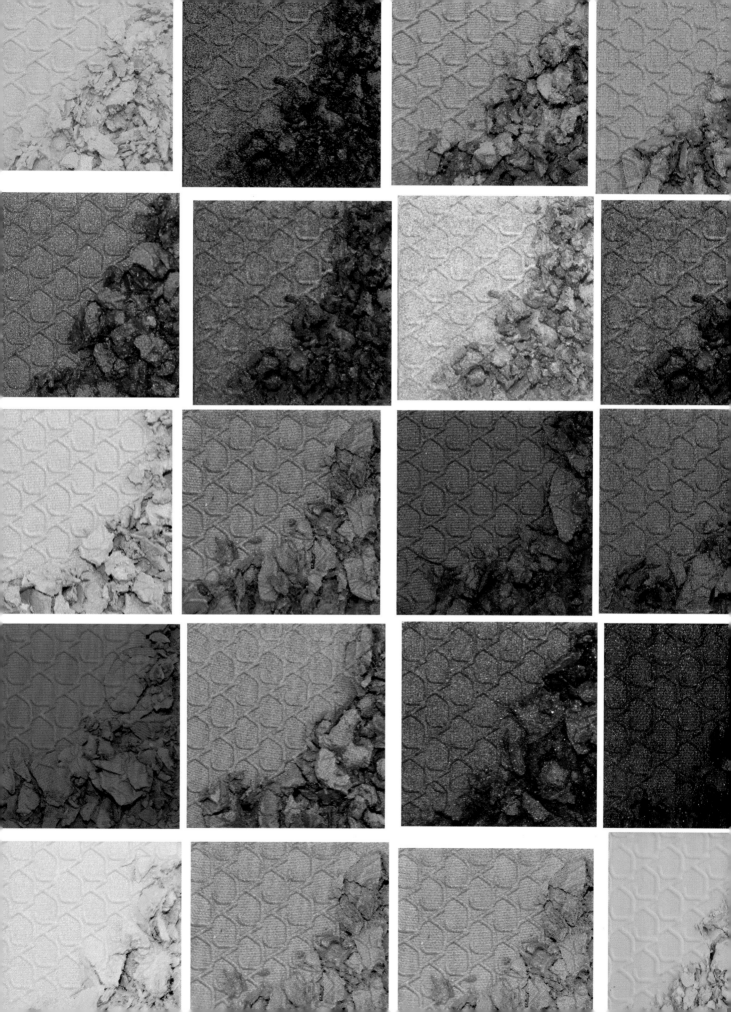

HOT-WEATHER MAKE-UP

Summer make-up is relaxed and natural, with less structure and polish. It's all about creating a sunkissed look, using warm tones to flatter tan skin.

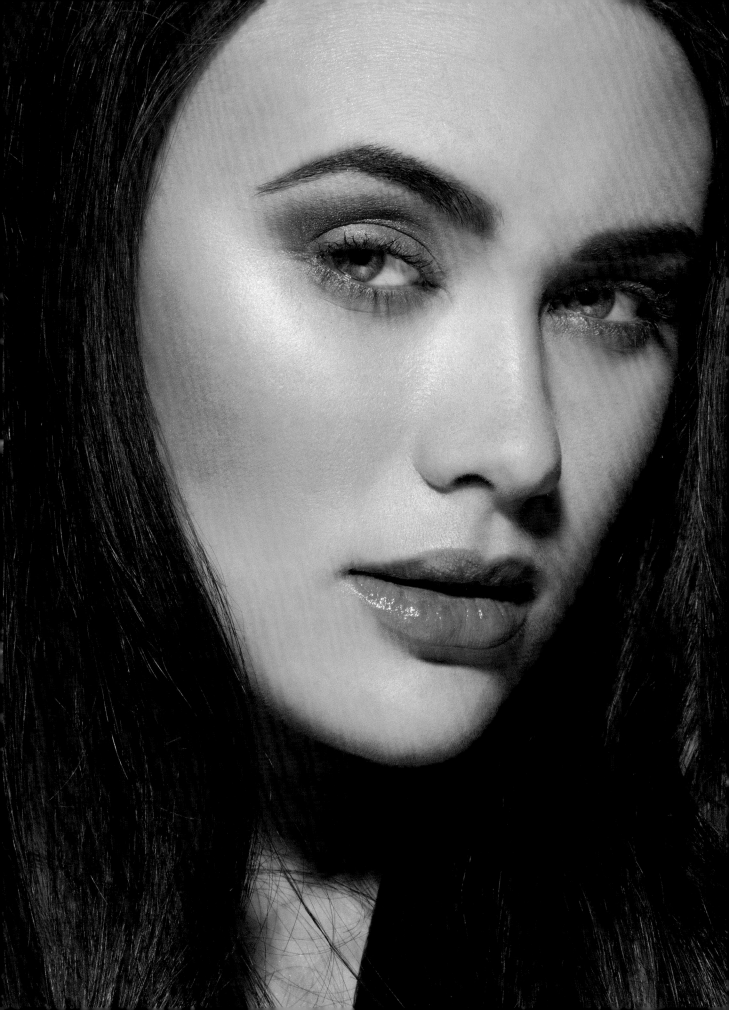

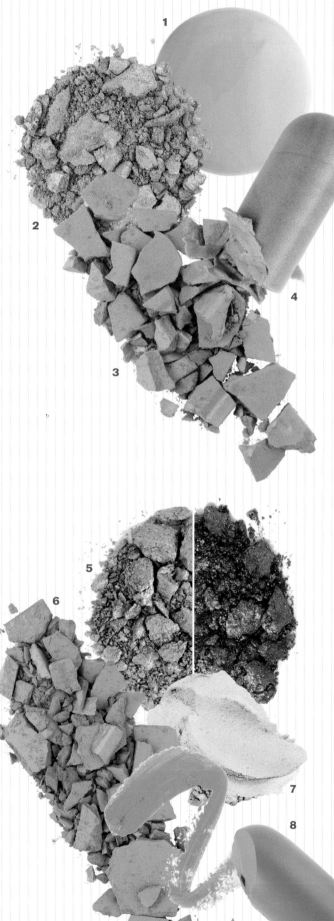

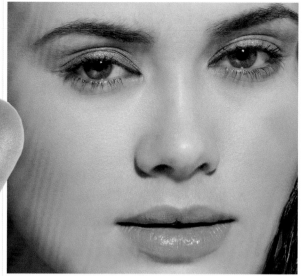

1 Apply high-SPF tinted moisturizer to even out the skin tone and provide light coverage.

2 Keep the eyes simple with a wash of shimmery powder eyeshadow in a taupe-gold color and a coat of black lash tint.

3 Give the apples of the cheeks a lovely warm glow with pinky apricot blush.

4 Use tinted lip balm during the day for an easy soft and pretty look.

5 At night, add definition to the lash lines and sockets with gold and bronze eyeshadows.

6 Accentuate the hollows of the cheeks with warm matte bronzer for more definition.

7 Add subtle highlights with radiance cream.

8 Apply satin lipstick in a rich coral pink.

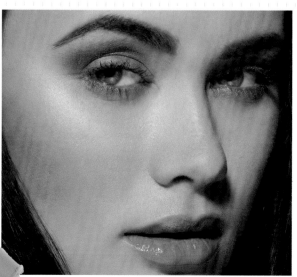

We tend to wear less make-up in the summer. When it's hot we wear fewer clothes, so more skin is exposed, making us feel healthy, free, and natural, and our approach to make-up reflects this. The main aim is to accentuate a healthy glow and highlight any natural tan. Freckles that come out in the sun are hard to cover, so it is preferable to keep any products on your face to the bare minimum. Keep your eyebrows tidy but not overly made-up: think natural beauty.

PALE SKIN
Anyone with pale skin can wear lovely soft pinks and pastel colors on the eyes. Equally, you can wear bright, vibrant lipsticks in shades of coral or fuchsia.

OLIVE SKIN
If your skin has yellow undertones, stay away from greens and yellows that will accentuate this; peach, copper, and bronze tones will help to brighten up the skin. Coral and orange lipsticks will look great on you.

DEEP SKIN
The darker shades of bronze, gold, berry, pomegranate, and bright pink are all really flattering, with gold-toned bronzers and lightly shimmering gold highlighter. Stay away from anything that has a grayness to it, such as blues, some purples, and grays.

Sunkissed skin

As your skin tone warms up naturally with exposure to the sun, you will probably need to go one or two shades deeper with your foundation or tinted moisturizer. This is when your color-mixing skills come into play (see page 23).

If the heat makes your skin excessively oily, use a primer with a silicone base that will help to absorb the oils. Mineral powder foundation or liquid foundation formulated to control oil are also good solutions.

Never put bronzer on bare skin—it will look awful. Bronzer looks most flattering on a flawless face and if you put it over blemishes, freckles, or unevenness, it will highlight them.

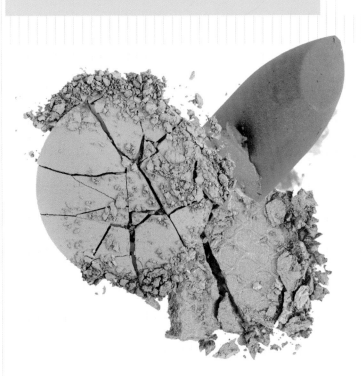

PRETTY PALETTE

Depending on how warm your skin tone is, you can either go for bright or pastel colors, or the warm golden hues of apricot and terracotta. Coral shades come around every summer without fail—it's a color you would never wear in the colder months but it is perfect for the brighter vibe of summer. Now is certainly the time to try out more vibrant lipsticks.

Simple washes of color eyeshadow work well in the summer. It's an easy way to experiment with new shades, such as pastels or aqua, and the result is suitably relaxed and low-key. I'm not a fan of high-shimmer textures because the skin tends to be naturally more sweaty. Soft pearl finishes are always flattering and easy to blend.

Dusty pinks, warm browns, and apricots all work well on the cheeks. If you're wearing a highlighter, opt for one with a golden tone.

COLD-WEATHER MAKE-UP

Much like winter clothes, cold-weather skincare is all about protection from the elements. Winter make-up tends to be less dewy and fresh-faced, with looks that are more structured and contoured.

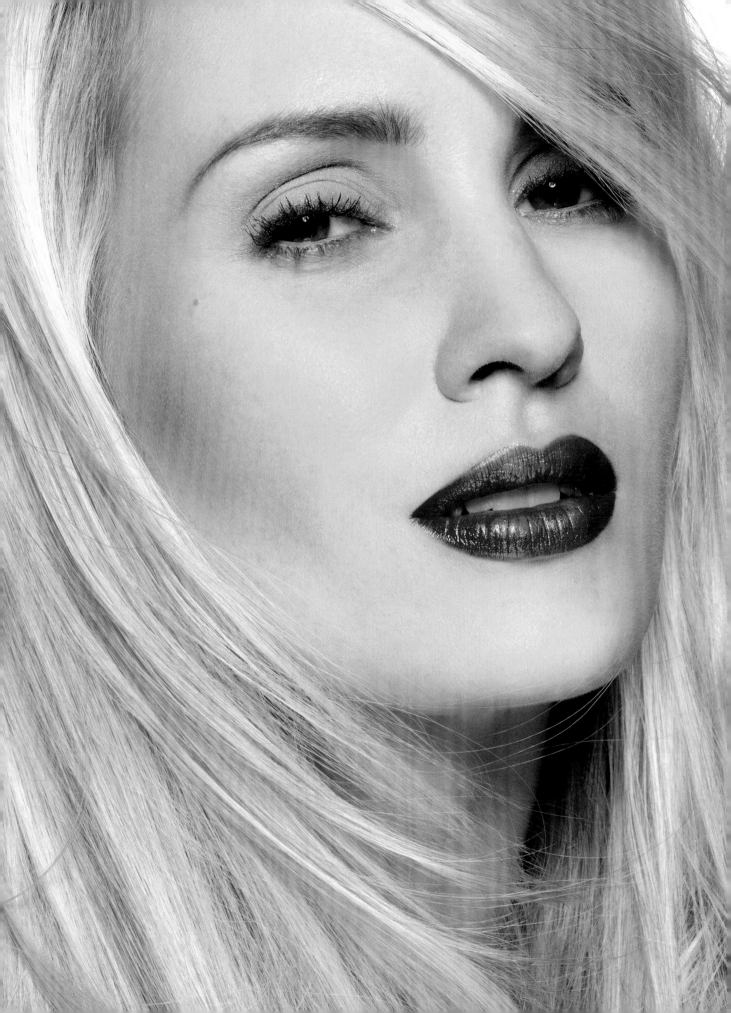

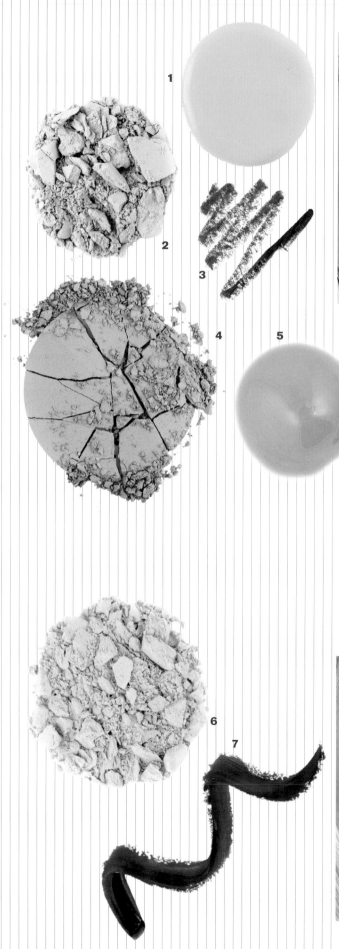

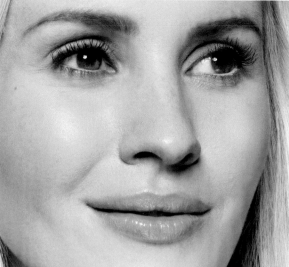

1 As winter skin dehydrates easily, use a hydrating primer over the face and eyelids, then even out the skin with liquid foundation.

2 Apply a cool nude powder eyeshadow as a simple colorwash over the eyelids.

3 Work gunmetal eyeliner into the roots of the lashes and blend. Use a nude pencil to fill in the waterlines to brighten the eyes, apply black mascara, and fill in the brows.

4 For a natural look, brush the cheeks lightly with a nude blush to add subtle warmth.

5 Keep the lips soft and natural with a light gloss in cool-toned petal pink.

6 At night, blend the eyeliner so it is really soft and apply a warm nude colorwash to the eyes.

7 Apply cool-toned bright red satin lipstick with a lip brush to create a precise shape.

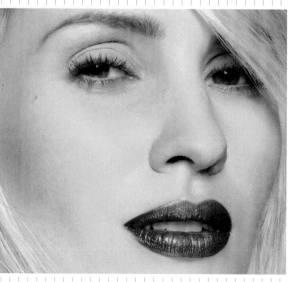

Winter is harsh on the skin, blasting it with freezing wind and rain and then exposing it to the drying atmosphere of centrally heated homes and offices. Broken capillaries can be caused by windburn and sudden changes in temperature; dehydration, flakiness, and chapped lips are also common problems. Keeping the skin moisturized, hydrated, and nourished is paramount.

Luminous skin

If you are using a thick face cream, make sure it has been fully absorbed by the skin before you put primer or foundation on top, otherwise it will just sit on the surface and not sink into the skin giving the natural finish you want.

I am a huge fan of primer, so I use one all year round—a radiance-boosting formulation is ideal for winter when skin often looks lackluster. For the same reason, I use a foundation with more luminosity, such as my Mineral Skin Nourishing Tint. Skin can sometimes be flaky in cold weather, so be careful if you use powder foundation, as it will accentuate any dryness.

Everything becomes duller in the winter, so pale skin tends to look pasty, olive skin appears sallow, and deep skin can look ashen. Counteract this by "lifting" and brightening the skin, using cream foundations, skin illuminators, and highlighters. Dark circles or blemishes will become more noticeable when the skin is paler. The good news is that you can get away with wearing more make-up, such as color correctors and concealer, to cover up any problems, as you are mostly seen in artificial light at this time of year, which is less harsh than daylight.

You always want a healthy glow, so blush is still an important part of cold-weather make-up. Winter doesn't mean you have to put away your bronzer, either, but make sure it is very subtle—only one shade darker than your skin—and has a matte finish to give a soft warmth to the face rather than a golden glow.

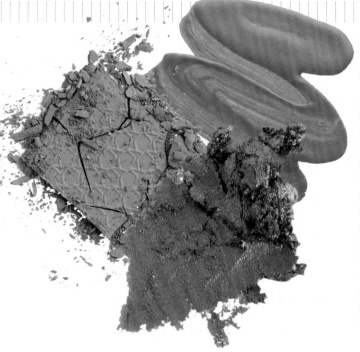

RICH PALETTE

I like looking at the colors found in nature. Deep berry shades come to the fore for cheeks and lips in the winter months. Eyeshadows go muddier and less pearlized, in richer shades of brown, gray, olive, plum, and eggplant. Colors are dusty and earthy—far from the vibrancy of summer's hues.

Powder finishes and matte textures are more fitting for winter and can be used for extensive blending, sculpting and contouring. Frosty shadows should be avoided, as they look too artificial. Brows are more defined, giving the entire effect more polish.

You can be more dramatic with the eyes and the mouth, with creamy hydrating lipsticks in deeper colors. Using a stain underneath a lipstick is a good way to increase its color intensity.

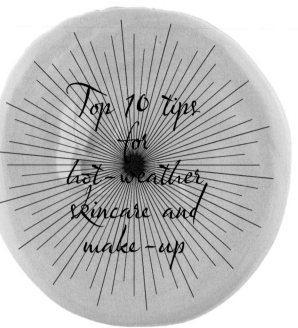

Top 10 tips for hot-weather skincare and make-up

1

Always use a higher factor SPF during the summer and reapply it regularly when you are outside for any length of time.

2

Include an antioxidant-rich serum in your skincare regime to help repair and protect.

3

Even out the skin tone with a lighter foundation or tinted moisturizer for sheer, veil-like coverage.

4

Use a lighter, less greasy moisturizer, especially during the day when your skin is likely to sweat more.

5

Use a creamy oil-based cleanser or mild Dove beauty bar to get rid of all traces of sweat and sunscreen without stripping the skin of its natural oils.

6

If you are wearing a vibrant color on the lips, wear less color on the eyes for a low-key vibe.

7

Make sure your lipstick is hydrating or wear balm underneath—choose one with SPF for extra protection.

8

Keep beach make-up simple—just a lick of waterproof mascara or lash tint, lip balm, and gloss—and get a spray tan before you go away to take the edge off your winter pallor.

9

Keep a pack of oil-blotting papers in your purse to tone down shine without adding more product.

10

Matte or soft pearl bronzing powder is made for the summer. Ensure the skin is flawless and lightly powdered, then brush the bronzer over the cheekbones, forehead, bridge of the nose, chin, and collarbones.

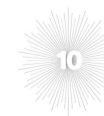

Top 10 tips for cold-weather skincare and make-up

1 Exfoliate regularly to slough off the dull surface layer. This reveals brighter new skin and helps to prevent any dry or flaky patches.

2 Swap serum for richer facial oil during the winter months to keep skin supple and smooth.

3 Use a richer, more nourishing face cream, but if you find this clogs up your skin, save it for nighttime and use a lighter moisturizer in the morning.

4 If you suffer from dehydrated skin, add Hyaluronic Acid drops to your moisturizer to boost hydration levels.

5 Don't put away the SPF—even weak winter sun contains harmful UV rays, so use a minimum of Factor 30.

6 Use a waxy lip balm to protect and nourish and help prevent dry, cracked lips. Keep balms in your purse, in your car, at work, in every room.

7 Stay away from any make-up in the orange color family and choose cooler pinks and richer earthy or berry shades.

8 If cold weather makes your eyes water, use a waterproof mascara or lash tint.

9 Always wear hand and nail cream to keep exposed hands protected and prevent them from drying out in the cold.

10 Richer cream foundation will provide better protective coverage for sensitized winter skin. Choose one with nourishing, radiance-boosting ingredients.

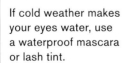

stop

the clock

One of the symptoms of modern living is that no one has time for anything. We are constantly rushing and multitasking to keep on top of our home, family, work and social lives.

Amid all this busyness, taking the time to put on make-up can seem like a luxury and often comes pretty low down on our list of priorities. However, it doesn't have to—there are some really great make-up looks for everything from work to parties that can be achieved in no time at all.

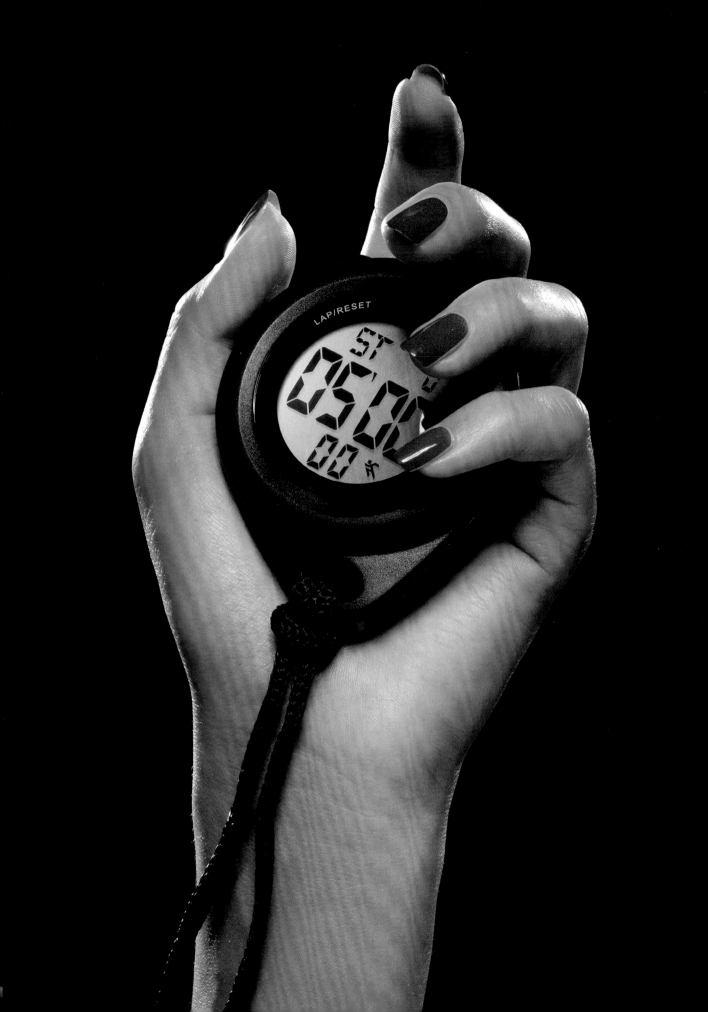

PERFECT
SKIN IN AN
INSTANT

When you are really pressed for time, just focus on perfecting your skin. Good skin instantly makes you look younger and less tired. It will make all the difference to how you look and feel.

When you don't have time to apply full make-up, four skin-perfecting products that will correct and enhance your complexion are all you need to achieve great skin in an instant. Redness, blemishes, and dark undereye shadows, which are such common complaints, can all be neutralized with my exclusive Citrus Color Corrector, while an apricot hue brightens and evens out the skin tone. A radiance cream adds essential luminosity and highlights to the skin— especially on cheekbones and browbones—while a multipurpose berry-colored tint gives a youthful flush to both lips and cheeks. The end result is a beautiful natural-looking complexion.

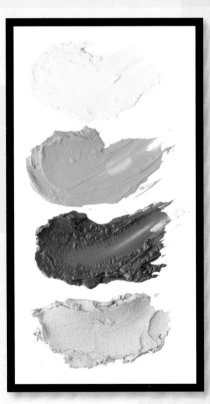

LEFT, top to bottom

Citrus color corrector combines yellow, to correct blue and purple undertones around the eye area, and green, to neutralize any red tones and blemishes.

Apricot color corrector neutralizes, brightens, and evens out the skin tone, especially around the eyes.

Berry lip and cheek tint, applied sparingly on the cheeks and lips, gives a natural, healthy flush.

Radiance cream, applied to areas that would naturally catch the light, defines and highlights the contours of the face.

If you only have time to do one thing, concentrate on your skin. Even out the skin tone and make it flawless and radiant.

Application

Use a synthetic brush or the pad of your fingers to press the cream color correctors into the skin with firm pats. Use a twisting motion to ensure you are not wiping it on and then off again.

1 Apply the Citrus Color Corrector first to cover up any blemishes, redness, or dark circles under the eyes. Pay particular attention to the areas around the nose, mouth, and under the lower lash line.

2 Use a brightening apricot color corrector to even out the skin tone and neutralize the citrus cream. You can apply it over your eyelids to provide a light natural coverage.

3 Blend a little radiance cream along the browbones, cheekbones, and bridge of the nose—anywhere that would naturally catch the light.

4 Blend the berry tint onto the apples of the cheeks and the lips. Apply it sparingly for a natural look.

5 Make sure all the edges are blended well and, if you wish, set with a dusting of fine translucent powder.

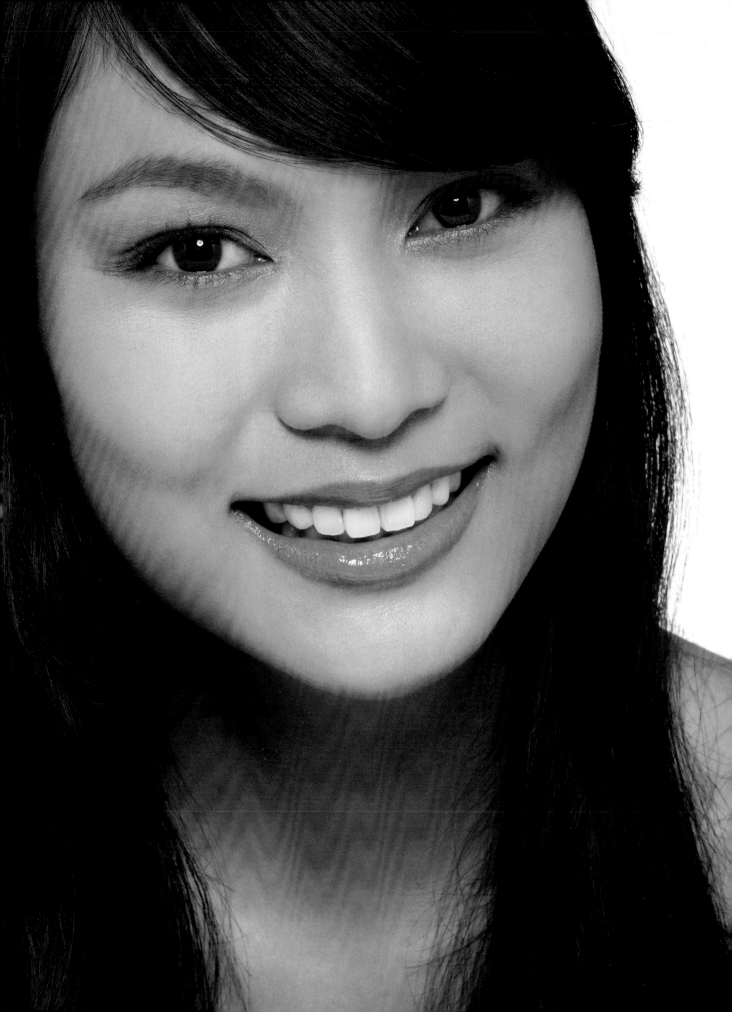

5 MINUTE MAKE-UP FOR LUNCH

When you are meeting friends for lunch, you want to look good, but as though you haven't had to try too hard. As daylight is harsh, less is definitely more with regard to make-up, so use products with sheer textures and soft luminosity to give a flawless finish with very light coverage—the skin should look fresh and glowing. Only use powder if you really need it to eliminate excess shine—on the T-zone, for example.

Look effortlessly radiant, with soft, natural colors, great skin, a little definition on the eyes, and a hydrated plump mouth.

Eyes

1 Brush the brows into shape and fill in any gaps with a matching powder, to make them look full.

2 Frame the eyes with brown eyeliner along the upper lash line, working it into the roots of the lashes and blending it up for a soft finish.

3 Blend rose-gold powder eyeshadow over the eyelids and above the crease. This is incredibly flattering, feminine, and natural. Apply a little on the lower lash line, blending it from the inner corner toward the outer corner, to brighten the eyes.

4 Curl the lashes—this is always important, especially if you have straight lashes, as it really opens up the eyes—then apply mascara.

Face

5 Apply a tinted moisturizer to even out the skin tone and create a flawless base in the most natural way. Use concealer if you need to cover up any blemishes.

6 Blend a little cream highlighter along the cheekbones and browbones to make the skin look really alive.

7 Use a pomegranate-colored cream blush, which blends to a sheer finish on tinted moisturizer. Apply it to the apples of the cheeks with your finger or a synthetic blush brush and blend it out to the hairline for a subtle healthy flush.

Lips

8 Add a slick of coral gloss to give your lips a warm color and a light shine.

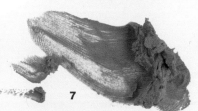

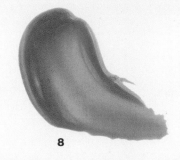

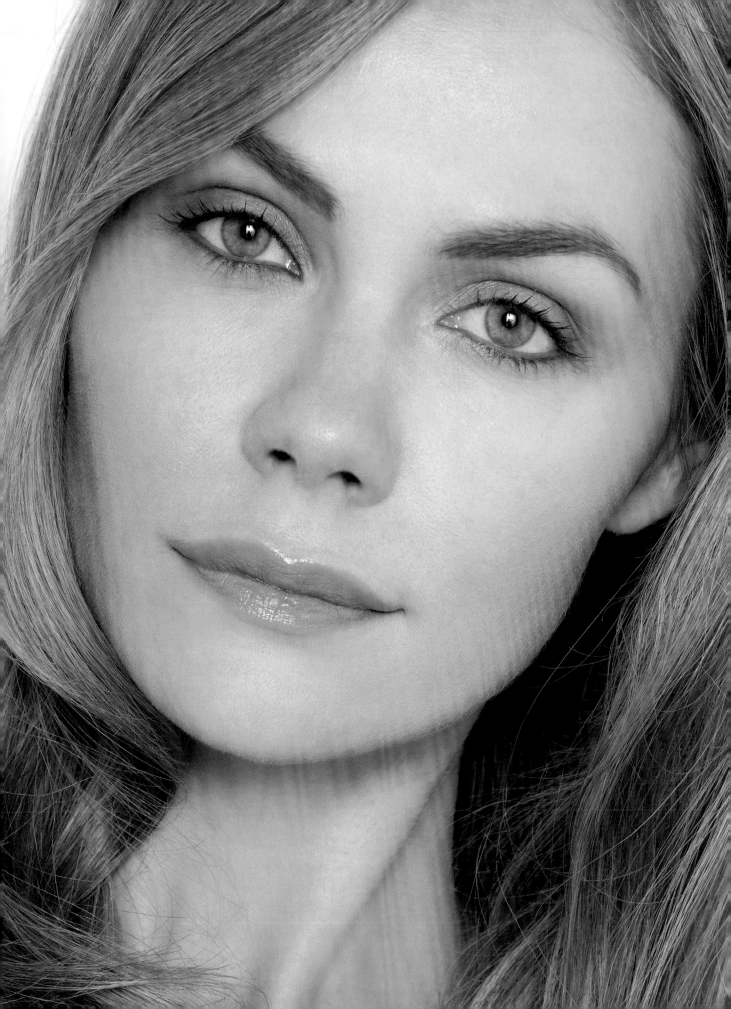

Make-up for the workplace needs to be subtle, enhancing your features in a natural way and making you look polished and professional.

The aim of any make-up that you wear to work is to empower you by boosting your confidence in the knowledge that you look your best. Neat, groomed brows are key, so pluck any stray hairs to maintain the shape before defining them. Skin has to be perfect—clean, flawless, and radiant, as though you've had eight hours sleep. Stick with matte or soft pearl products and don't use anything that is shiny or iridescent, as artificial office lighting will highlight it too much.

Eyes

1 Using an angled brush and a matte powder that matches your eyebrows, draw a sharp line right under the brow to define the shape. Then blend the color up into the brow with light feathery strokes. This gives a strong shape but with a soft, natural finish.

2 Prep and prime the eyelids to give a longer-lasting base and to eliminate any redness, which will make you look tired.

3 Brush light gray eyeshadow over the entire lid. Define the socket with a darker gray, blending it out and focusing on the outer corners. Use a soft brush so you can blend as you apply—the primer makes blending quicker and holds the pigment, so you can apply less eyeshadow.

4 Apply gunmetal eyeliner along the upper lash line, working it into the roots of the lashes to make them look fuller. Dot eyeliner along the roots of the lower lashes and blend it out to make them look thicker without creating a hard line.

5 Apply mascara to the top lashes only.

Face

6 Apply primer over the face to ensure a smooth base that lasts all working day. If you have oily skin, use an oil-absorbing primer for a matte finish. Blend liquid foundation over the areas that need it, especially beneath the eyes and around the nose and mouth. Use concealer as necessary to cover up dark circles or blemishes.

7 Mattify the face with a light dusting of translucent powder.

8 Using a medium blush brush, apply matte bronzer under the cheekbones to sculpt them. The powder underneath will soften the color and give a subtle finish.

Lips

9 Finish with a soft pink lipstick with a creamy hydrating formula that is not too glossy but not too pigmented. I used my Glosstick in Sugar Cane to give soft color without too much of a statement; it is very moisturizing and quick to apply.

5 MINUTE MAKE-UP FOR A DATE

This is a fresh, pretty, innocent look that is feminine and attractive without being too vampy or overtly sexy.

When you are going on a date, aim to look your best without appearing too made-up—you want to give the illusion that you look like this all the time. No masks and no false advertising. Skin must be clear, fresh, and naturally radiant with a healthy flush to the cheeks, eyes should look bright and sparkly, and lips should be soft and kissable. Play up your best feature: if you have a big smile and a great mouth, emphasize your lips and wear lots of gloss; if you have gorgeous eyes, bring the focus onto them.

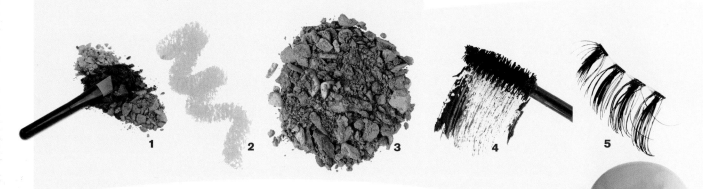

Eyes

1 Tidy the brows and fill in any gaps with matching brow powder and an angled brush to frame the face.

2 Prime the eyes to get rid of redness and create a base for the eyeshadow.

3 Blend a soft pearl eyeshadow in a light natural tone, such as a rosy gold, over the entire lid to brighten and subtly define the eyes. Blend a little along the lower lash line for a soft finish.

4 Coat the top and bottom lashes with lots of black mascara.

5 Add corner lashes to open up and elongate the eyes.

Face

6 Apply a light foundation only where you need it to even out the skin tone and cover up any flaws.

7 Blend cream highlighter along the cheekbones for extra radiance.

8 Blend a little lip and cheek tint into the apples of the cheeks for a really natural sheer flush.

9 Apply the lip and cheek tint to the lips, too, for a natural stain, and brush a rose-pink gloss on top.

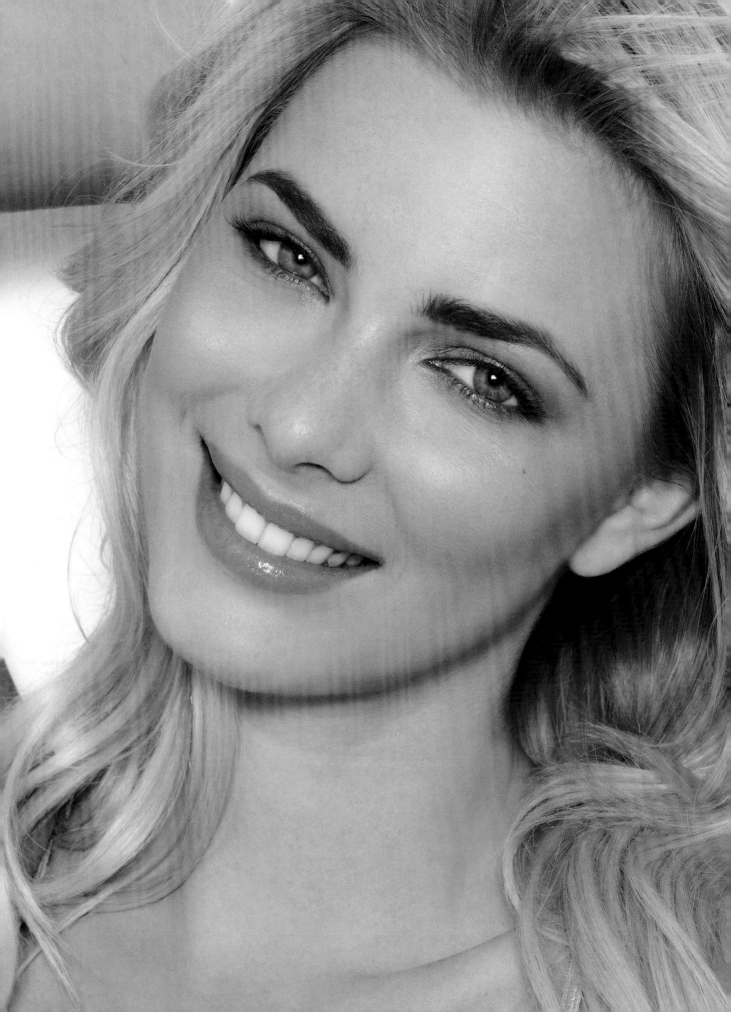

5 MINUTE MAKE-UP FOR A PARTY

Party make-up is about creating impact, and here the focus is brought onto the eyes with vibrant blue eyeliner.

Parties are the time to have fun with statement make-up. Bright colors, glitter liners, metallic pigment, and fashion lashes with feathers or jewels are great options—though not all at once. Nothing in this look steals the limelight from the eyes, which are made to pop with an accent of color and corner lashes. Make-up can be stronger when it is going to be seen in artificial light, so you can use more foundation set with powder for longer-lasting flawless coverage and a stronger powder blush to define the cheeks.

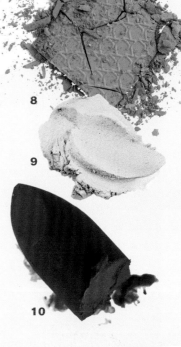

Eyes

1 Prep and prime the eyes to create a neutral base and make them look fresh and bright.

2 Apply an amethyst silk crayon along the top lash line, making the line quite thick and defined. Blend the same color along the lower lash line, using a smudger or brush to soften it.

3 Apply blue glitter gel liner along the upper lash line, making the line thickest in the middle of the eye and tapering it out at the inner and outer corners. Ensure both eyes are symmetrical.

4 Curl the lashes and apply a coat of black mascara.

5 Add corner lashes and another coat of mascara for extra drama.

Face

6 Apply foundation and blend it well for a flawless finish.

7 Set the make-up with light-reflecting powder to eliminate shine.

8 Blush can be stronger than normal for long-lasting definition. Apply powder blush with a natural-bristle brush, building up the color gradually and blending it well from the apples of the cheeks out toward the hairline.

9 Blend a little highlighter along the cheekbones and browbones.

Lips

10 Apply a rich berry-colored lipstick and blot it with a tissue for a softer finish. Dab a little clear gloss onto the back of your hand and apply it over the lipstick with a lip brush.

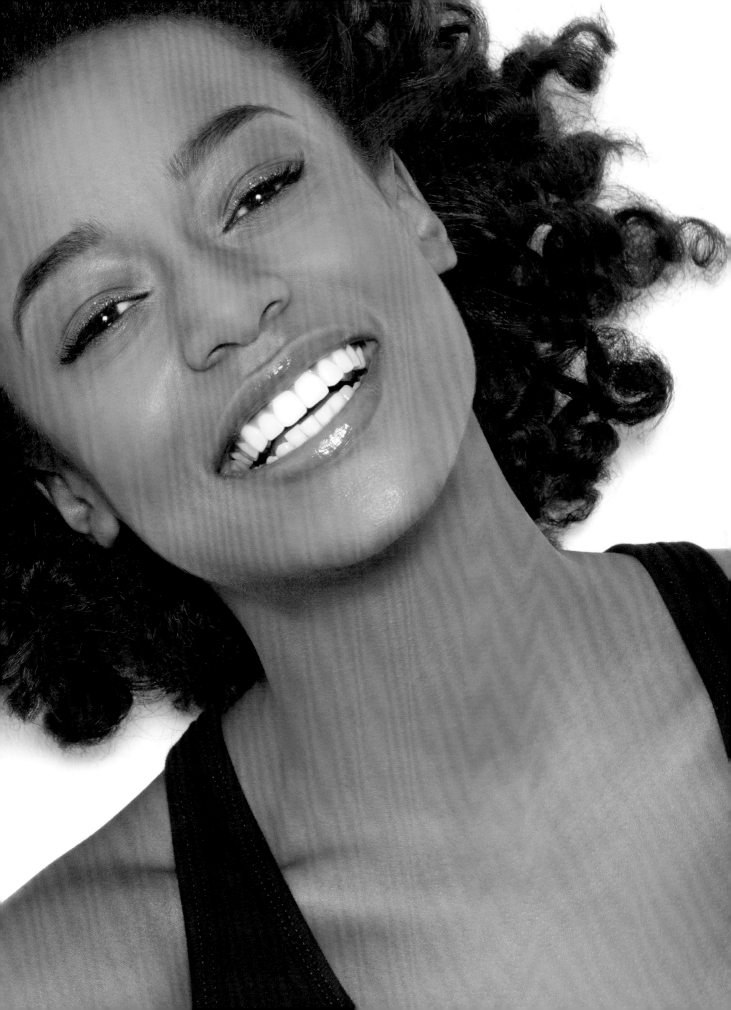

JEMMA'S FAVORITES

FACIAL SKINCARE PRODUCTS

Cleansers
Dove Beauty Bar

Eye Make-up Removers
Dior Duo Magique Duo-Phase
  Eye Makeup Remover
L'Oréal De-Maq Expert

Exfoliators
Sarah Chapman Skinesis
  Overnight Exfoliating Booster

Daily Moisturizers
Sarah Chapman Skinesis
  Dynamic Defence SPF 15
SteamCream

Night Moisturizers
Elemis Pro-Collagen
  Marine Cream
Sarah Chapman Skinesis
  Overnight Facial

Eye Creams
Yon Ka Phyto-Contour Eye
  Firming Cream
Zelens Intensive Triple-Action
  Eye Cream

Hydrating Masks
Sarah Chapman Skinesis
  Instant Miracle Mask
Sisley Express Flower Gel

Facial Oils/Serums
RODIN Olio Lusso Luxury
  Face Oil
SkinCeuticals C E Ferulic
SkinCeuticals Hyaluronic Acid

Facial SPFs
Elave Daily Skin Defence
  SPF 30+
JĀSÖN Facial Natural
  Sunblock SPF20
La Roche-Posay Anthelios XL
  SPF 50+
Neutrogena Pure and Free

Lip Balm
Jemma Kidd Make Up School
  Hi-Shine Hydrating Glosstick
  SPF 15

Lucas Pawpaw Ointment
NUXE Baume Prodigieux
  Lèvres

BODY PRODUCTS

Hand Cream
L'Occitane Shea Butter
  Hand Cream

Exfoliators
Jo Malone Vitamin E Body
  Treatment Scrub

Moisturizers
NEOM Luxury Organic
  Bath Oils
L'Occitane Shea Butter
  Ultra Rich Body Cream
Pure Coconut Oil—best
  body oil

Body Shimmer
JK Jemma Kidd Show Stopper
  Year-Round Body Glow

MAKE-UP AND TOOLS

EYES

Brows
Jemma Kidd Make Up School
  Brow Perfector Shape and
  Lift Duo

Eye Pencil
Jemma Kidd Make Up School
  Define Stay-Put Eyeliner

Liquid Eyeliners
Bobbi Brown Long-Wear
  Gel Eyeliner

Powder Eyeshadows
Chanel Ombre Essentielle
JK Jemma Kidd I-Design
  Eye Colour

Lash Curler
Shu Uemura Eyelash Curler

Mascara
Jemma Kidd Make Up School
  Lash Xtension Volume
  Mascara

FACE

Primer
JK Jemma Kidd Instant Lift
  Skin Perfecting Primer

Tinted Moisturizer
Jemma Kidd Make Up School
  Mineral Skin Nourishing Tint
  SPF 20

Liquid Foundations
Jemma Kidd Make Up School
  Light as Air SPF 18
Make Up For Ever HD High
  Definition Foundation

Loose Powder
Jemma Kidd Make Up School
  Bio-Mineral Perfecting Powder
Laura Mercier Secret
  Brightening Powder

Undereye concealers
JK Jemma Kidd Mannequin
  Skin Illuminating Brightener
  & Concealer Duo

Skin Illuminator
JK Jemma Kidd Mannequin
  Skin Complexion Enhancer

Blemish Concealer
Laura Mercier Secret Camouflage

Complexion Enhancers
Jemma Kidd Make Up School
  Pro Skin Rescue Bio Complex
  Veil SPF15

Highlighters
Jemma Kidd Make Up School
  Dewy Glow All Over
  Radiance Crème

Powder Blushes
Jemma Kidd Make Up School
  Tailored Colour Powder
  Blush Duo
Nars Blush

Cream Blushes
Bobbi Brown Pot Rouge for
  Lips & Cheeks
Jemma Kidd Make Up School
  Blushwear Crème Cheek
  Colour

LIPS

Lip liner
Jemma Kidd Make Up School
  Shape and Shade Liner and
  Lip Fill

Lipsticks
Guerlain Kiss Kiss
Jemma Kidd Make Up School
  Ultimate Lipstick Duo

Lip gloss
Jemma Kidd Make Up School
  Hi Shine Silk Touch Lipgloss

NAIL VARNISHES

Chanel Nail Colour
OPI Nail Polish

ORGANIC MAKE-UP AND SKINCARE BRANDS

Aesop
Aveda
Bare Minerals
Dr Hauschka—for foundation
  and bronzer
Elave
Green People—for lipstick
JĀSÖN
Living Nature—for mascara
Nvey Eco
Origins
Ren
The Organic Pharmacy
There Must Be A Better
  Way—for lip balm

BRANDS AND PRODUCTS FOR PROBLEM SKIN

Clinique Pore Minimizer
Clinique Redness Solutions
Coverblend—cosmetic
  camouflage
Covermark—cosmetic
  camouflage

Dermablend—cosmetic
camouflage
Dr Hauschka Rose Day Cream—
for sensitive rosacea-prone skin
Elave—for sensitive skin and
sufferers of dermatitis,
psoriasis, and eczema
Prescriptives—for custom-
blended foundation and powder
Proactiv—for acne-prone skin

TREATMENTS

London

Aglaia Hernandez Kortis at
Natureworks—for massage
(+44 (0)20 7629 2927;
www.natureworks.net)
Sarah Chapman—for facials
(www.sarahchapman.net)
Shavata Brow Studio
(www.shavata.co.uk)
Spa NK
(www.uk.spacenk.com)
Strip Waxing Bar
(www.stripwaxbar.com)
Una Brennan—for facials
(+44 (0)20 7313 9835)
Urban Retreat Spa at Harrods
(www.urbanretreat.co.uk/
harrods)
Vanda Serrador at Urban Skin—
for facials and body treatments
(www.urban-skin.com)

New York

Ashley Javier Parlor—
for haircut and color
(+1 (0) (212) 252 8794;
www.ashleyjavierparlor.com)
Bliss Spa
(www.blissworld.com/spa)
Dr Amy Wexler Dermatology
(www.dramywechsler.com)
Dr David Colbert, New York
Dermatology Group
(www.nydermatolgoygroup.
com)

VITAMINS AND SUPPLEMENTS

BioCare Vitamin C 1000
Boiron Oscillococcinum—
for colds and flu
Comvita Pure Manuka Honey
Lozengers—for sore throats
Floradix Floravital Yeast & Gluten
Free Liquid Iron Formula

Manuka Health Manuka Honey
MGO 100—for sore throats
Solgar Chelated Magnesium
Solgar Vitamin-B Complex
Solgar Elderberry Extract—
for colds
Spatone 100% Natural Iron
Supplement
Symprove—live probiotic
Udo's Choice Ultimate Oil
Blend Omega 3-6-9 Oil
Capsules
Weleda Ferrum Phos
Homeopathic Tablets—
for colds

FURTHER READING

The Green Smoothies Diet
by Robyn Openshaw-Pay
Green Smoothie Revolution
by Victoria Boutenko
The Healthy Green Drink Diet
by Jason Manheim
*The Juice Master: Turbo-
charge Your Life in 14 Days*
by Jason Vale
The Mind-Beauty Connection
by Amy Wechsler, MD

STOCKISTS

For JK Jemma Kidd range
www.jemmakidd.com
www.target.com (USA)
www.asos.com (UK)
**For Jemma Kidd Make Up
School range**
www.jemmakidd.com
www.lookfantastic.com
www.feelunique.com
**For information on
professional make-up
courses and non-
professional make-up
workshops, visit**
www.jemmakidd.com
+44 (0)844 800 2636

Aesop
www.beautyexpert.co.uk
Allergy Research Group
www.allergyresearchgroup.com
Aveda
www.aveda.co.uk
Bare Minerals
www.bareminerals.co.uk
BioCare
www.biocare.co.uk

Bionutri
www.bionutri.co.uk
Bliss
www.blissworld.com
Bobbi Brown
www.bobbibrown.co.uk
Boiron
www.chelseahealthstore.com
Burt's Bees
www.burtsbees.com
Chanel
www.chanel.com
Clinique
www.clinique.co.uk
Comvita
www.comvita.co.uk
Coverblend
www.neostrata.com
Covermark
www.covermark.com
Dermablend
www.dermablend.co.uk
Dior
www.dior.com
Dove
www.dove.co.uk
Dr Hauschka
www.drhauschka.co.uk
Elave
www.elave.co.uk
Elemis
www.elemis.com
ELF
www.eyeslipsface.co.uk
Floradix Floravital
www.victoriahealth.com
Green People
www.greenpeople.co.uk
Guerlain
www.guerlain.com
JĀSÖN
www.jasonnaturalcare.co.uk
Jo Malone
www.jomalone.co.uk
La Roche-Posay
www.laroche-posay.co.uk
Laura Mercier
www.lauramercier.com
Living Nature
www.naturisimo.com
L'Occitane
www.uk.loccitane.com
L'Oréal
www.loreal.co.uk
Lucas Pawpaw
www.pawpawshop.co.uk
Make Up For Ever
www.makeupforever.com
Manuka Health
www.yourhealthfoodstore.co.uk

Nars
www.narscosmetics.co.uk
NEOM
www.neomorganics.com
Neutrogena
www.neutrogena.com
NUXE
www.nuxe.com
Nvey Eco
www.nveyeco.co.uk
Origins
www.origins.co.uk
OPI
www.opi.com
Prescriptives
www.prescriptives.co.uk
Proactiv
www.proactiv.co.uk
Ren
www.renskincare.com
RODIN Olio Lusso
www.oliolusso.com
Sarah Chapman
www.sarahchapman.net
Shu Uemura
www.spacenk.co.uk
SkinCeuticals
www.skinceuticals.co.uk
Sisley
www.sisley-cosmetics.co.uk
Solgar
www.solgar.com
Space NK Apothecary
www.uk.spacenk.com
Spatone
www.nelsonsnaturalworld.com
SteamCream
www.steamcream.co.uk
Symprove
www.symprove.com
The Organic Pharmacy
www.theorganicpharmacy.com
There Must Be A Better Way
www.theremustbeabetterway.
co.uk
Udo's Choice Oil
www.udoschoice.co.uk
Weleda
www.yourhealthfoodstore.co.uk
Yon Ka
www.feelunique.com
Zelens
www.zelens.com

INDEX

ACKNOWLEDGMENTS

Make-up artists
Jemma Kidd
Jodie Hazlewood
Miriam Jensen
Claire Woyton
Louise O'Neill
Hair stylists
Davide Barbieri
Marcia Lee
Art director and designer
Lawrence Morton
**Commissioning editor
and writer**
Zia Mattocks
Photographer
Vikki Grant
Digital operator
Karl Grant
Product photographer
Natasha Lewis
**Assistant product
photographer**
Kirsty McGill
Co-ordinator
Elisa Drummond

Models
Annaliese Dayes (Zone
    Models)
Bailee Roup (MOT Models)
Caroline Royce (Close Models)
Charlotte De Carle (Nevs
    Models)
Dara Bascara (Sandra
    Reynolds)
Hannah L (BMA Model
    Management)
Joanna Stubbs (Models 1)
Jona Jarvenpaa (Zone Models)
Joy (Models 1)
Juliana Aneli (Nevs Models)
Kajsa M (FM Agency)
Katja Zwara (MOT Models)
Louise R (BMA Model
    Management)

With thanks to
Alexandra Labbe Thompson,
Catherine Bailey, Jackie Haigh,
Abbey Campbell, and Alex
Longmore

Thanks to:
American Apparel
    store.americanapparel.co.uk/
Sarah Chapman
    Sarah Chapman Skinesis
    Clinic, 106 Draycott Avenue,
    London SW3 3AE
    +44 (0)20 7589 9585
    www.sarahchapman.net
Petronella Ravenshear
    Chelsea Nutrition, Smith
    Street, London SW3 4EE
    +44 (0)20 7730 8289
    www.chelseanutrition.com
Shavata Singh
    www.shavata.co.uk

Special thanks to:
Arthur Mornington, Mae
Wellesley, Darcy Wellesley,
Wendy Kidd, Kati St Clair,
Nadja Gydat, Kelvin Heard,
Sally Killingback, Amanda
Griggs, Golden Hummingbird,
Chinese Heritage.

This book wouldn't have been
possible without all of the hard
work and dedication from the
entire team. I would like to say
a huge thank you to Jacqui
Small, Zia Mattocks, Lawrence
Morton, Kerenza Swift, Lydia
Halliday, Jodie Hazlewood,
Miriam Jensen, Elisa
Drummond, Claire Woyton,
Louise O'Neil, David Barbieri,
Marcia Lee, Vikki Grant, Karl
Grant, Natasha Lewis, and
Kirsty McGill.

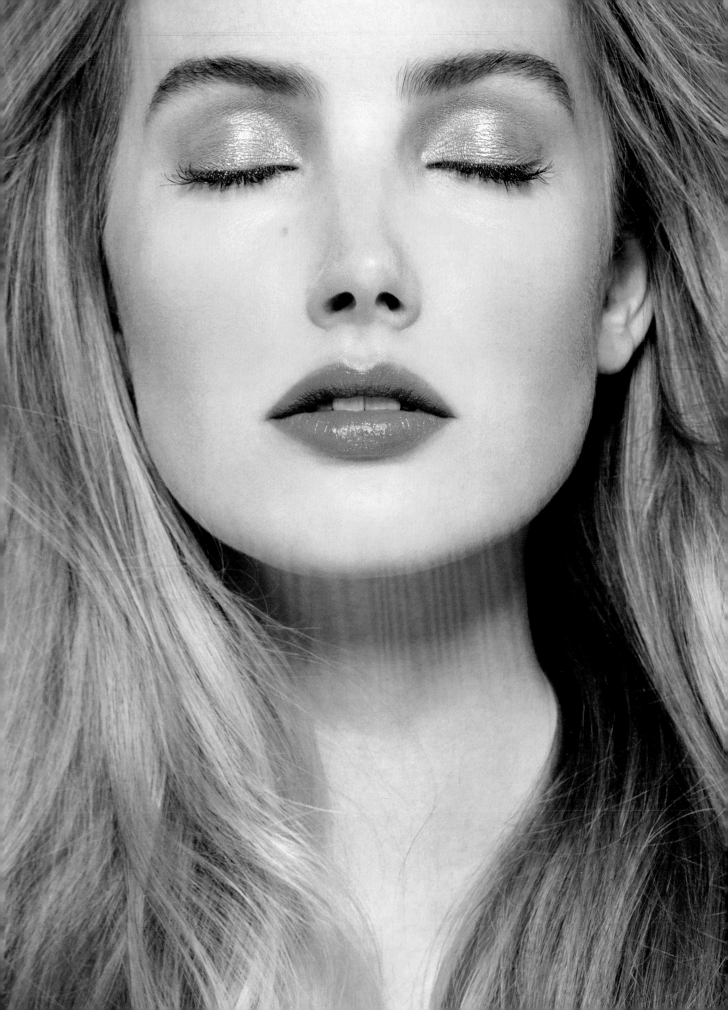

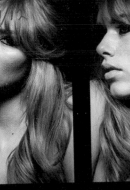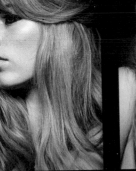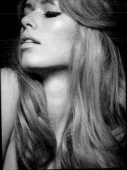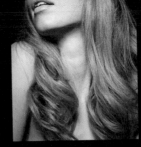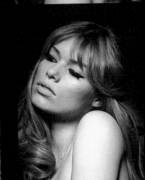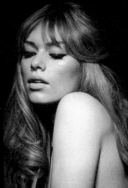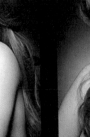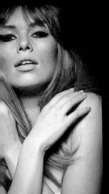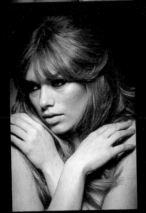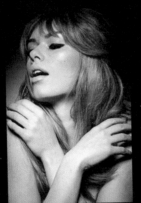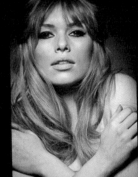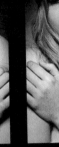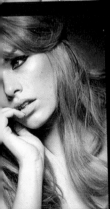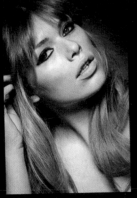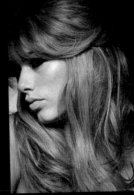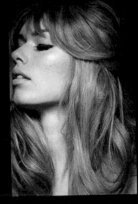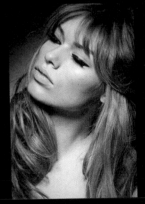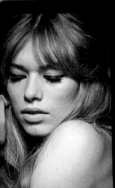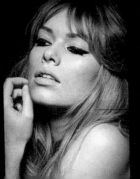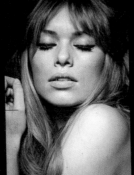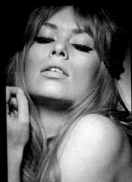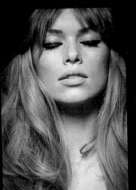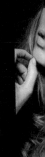